Ketogenic Meal Plan
for Beginners: An Easy, Low Carb, 5-Ingredient Cookbook

A Simple 30-Day Meal Plan for Quick Weight Loss

Anna Lane

© **Copyright 2020 - All rights reserved.**

The content contained within this book may not be reproduced, duplicated or transmitted without direct written permission from the author or the publisher.

Under no circumstances will any blame or legal responsibility be held against the publisher, or author, for any damages, reparation, or monetary loss due to the information contained within this book, either directly or indirectly.

Legal Notice:

This book is copyright protected. It is only for personal use. You cannot amend, distribute, sell, use, quote or paraphrase any part, or the content within this book, without the consent of the author or publisher.

Disclaimer Notice:

Please note the information contained within this document is for educational and entertainment purposes only. All effort has been executed to present accurate, up to date, reliable, complete information. No warranties of any kind are declared or implied. Readers acknowledge that the author is not engaged in the rendering of legal, financial, medical or professional advice. The content within this book has been derived from various sources. Please consult a licensed professional before attempting any techniques outlined in this book.

By reading this document, the reader agrees that under no circumstances is the author responsible for any losses, direct or indirect, that are incurred as a result of the use of the information contained within this document, including, but not limited to, errors, omissions, or inaccuracies.

Table of Contents

Author's Message 7
Chapter 1 9
How the Keto Diet Works 9
Chapter 2 11
Why Choose Keto? 11
Chapter 3 15
Where Do You Start? 15
Chapter 4 22
The Secret Ingredient 22
Calories 22
Exercise 25
Chapter 5 28
THE 30-Day KETO DIET MEAL PLAN TO LET YOU SUCCEED! 28

BREAKFAST 36
Vegetable Scrambled Eggs 36
Egg Muffin 38
Sausage and Fried Eggs 40
Boiled Eggs and Avocado Plate 42
Breakfast Patties 44
Bacon and Egg Breakfast Muffin 46
Spinach Egg Muffin 48
Cheese Omelet 50
Breakfast Egg Salad 52
Bacon and Egg Cup 54
Cheesy Avocado Egg Boat 56
Cauliflower Hash Browns 58
Bell Pepper Eggs 60
Cinnamon Muffin 62
Beef and Spinach Frittata 64
Eggs in Clouds 66
Bagel 68
Cream Cheese Pancake 70
Mozzarella and Garlic Waffles 72
Porridge 74
Jalapeno Waffle 76

Breakfast Vanilla Pudding 78
Waffles with Poached Eggs 80
Pumpkin Spiced Hemp Porridge 82
Breakfast Tuna Wrap 84
Beef Omelet Wrap 86
Peanut Butter Oatmeal 88
Cheesy Vegetable Frittata 90
Chicken and Bacon Pancake 92
Cheesy Garlic Bacon Knots 94

LUNCH 96

Cheese Muffin 96
Meat Muffin 98
Tuna Egg Boats 100
Stuffed Zucchini Boats 102
Lettuce Wraps 104
Creamy Broccoli Salad 106
Tuna Cakes 108
Spinach Stuffed Zucchini 110
Cider Chicken Thighs 112
Bacon Wrapped Asparagus 114
Beef Stuffed Avocado 116
Salmon Patties 118
Cheesy Zoodles 120
Taco Radish Wedges 122
Sweet and Spicy Brussel Sprouts 124
Paprika Chicken 126
Egg and Spinach Salad 128
Cheesy Cauliflower Soup 130
Spinach Salad with Feta Dressing 132
Lettuce and Avocado Rolls 134
Garlic Zoodles 136
Lime and Garlic Chicken Thighs 138
Tuna Salad 140
Cheesy Deviled Eggs with Avocado 142
Ranch Deviled Eggs 144
Caprese Salad 146
Marinara Deviled Egg 148
Asparagus and Tomato Salad 150

Pork and Egg Cup 152
Berries in Yogurt Cream 154

DINNER **156**
Shrimp and Bacon 156
Chili 158
Pumpkin Soup 160
Roasted Cauliflower Steaks 162
Bacon Wrapped Chicken 164
Teriyaki Chicken 166
Coconut Crusted Fish 168
Red Curry Glazed Fish 170
Beef and Broccoli 172
Cheesy Kale Patties 174
Chicken Nuggets 176
Broccoli and Cheese Soup 178
Cheddar Chicken 180
Tuna and Spinach Salad 182
Meatloaf 184
Pulled Chicken 186
Buttery Salmon 188
Salmon with Green Beans 190
Cream of Asparagus Soup 192
Chicken Salad 194
Bacon-Wrapped Salmon 196
Creamy Chicken Soup 198
Cheesy Chicken Stuffed Bell Pepper 200
Beef and Spinach Sliders 202
Basil Stuffed Chicken 204
Chicken and Coconut Curry 206
Herbed Steaks 208
Pork Cutlets 210
Pork Chops with Mushrooms 212
Cocoa Rubbed Pork 214

Conclusion 216

References 217

Author's Message

Starting on a new diet is never easy. Whether you're seeking to improve your general health, save yourself from obesity, or just shed some extra pounds in preparation for summer, dieting is a pain. But it doesn't always have to be! I've devoted years trying to lose weight. During my journey, dozens of fad diets came and went, so I spent thousands on equipment and specialized meal plans, all to no avail. That was, until a friend told me about this diet casually known as keto... To be honest, I thought they were crazy when they told me that the diet was based on eating primarily fatty foods. I even remember asking them, "If fat is so good for losing weight, then why do I still have this belly?" Ugh!

In retrospect, I was still skeptical even after they convinced me to join them. But I was determined, so I busily prepared myself for the diet. I removed all of the food I wasn't allowed to eat from my house, researched meal plans, bought the necessary ingredients, and determined my calorific needs. This readiness all took weeks because I had no idea where to start. Those hours of research and my subsequent success with keto greatly inspired me to write this book. I decided that I needed to introduce others to keto and help those in the same position. This book is everything you need to get started on your journey to a better you!

You won't need to spend weeks researching because everything you need is right here at your fingertips. First, you'll find a brief explanation of what keto is and how it works, but you'll also discover tips on how to get started, details on the science behind keto, and a breakdown on the benefits this diet has for you.

Now, no keto cookbook is complete without a long list of mouth-watering recipes. All the recipes included in these pages are familiar, affordable, and easy to prepare. Each one is tasty, healthy, and guaranteed to ensure your keto diet has some of the best home eating ever! You won't need to devote hours preparing ingredients, and you won't need to be a qualified chef to cook any of these meals. All you need is a few minutes from your busy day and an empty stomach to motivate you. Regardless of your work hours or busy home life, switching to keto can be a breeze with these simple recipes.

Eating habits are probably the hardest thing to change when switching diets; the way we eat is a big part of our lives. When switching to keto, it can be tough. To illustrate, that bowl of muesli or piece of toast you had for breakfast is no longer allowed, and that burger is no longer an appealing lunch option. But with a little help, your eating habits can be changed in a relaxed and stress-free manner. In this book, you'll access a month-long meal plan to guide you through your first weeks of keto dieting. The meal plan comes complete with reference pictures of each full meal, a nutritional breakdown of every dish, and a table of ingredients with scaling portions up to 8 people!

Chapter 1

How the Keto Diet Works

The keto diet is an incredibly effective form of a low-carb, high-fat diet. Fat tends to be a scary word when approaching diets, as almost all mainstream diets revolve around cutting out as much fat as possible. With the keto diet, fat is our friend. The vast majority of people rely on carbohydrates as their energy source, but in the keto diet we train our bodies to consume fat as our main source of energy.

The keto diet looks to convince our bodies to use a different type of fuel. Usually, we'd rely on glucose, which comes from carb heavy food. The main goal of the keto diet is to reach a stage of ketosis. Ketosis is a metabolic process in which our body burns through our fat reserves for energy, creating water-soluble acid molecules called ketone bodies (or ketones). Keep in mind, reaching ketosis can be tricky. To achieve a state of ketosis in our body, we need to ensure that we consume less than 50 grams of carbs per day, and some experts even recommend as low as 20 grams. It may take up to a week for your body to reach ketosis, even with a low-carb intake, so patience is key.

A common misconception about the keto diet is that it doesn't provide the glucose needed to sustain crucial parts of our brain. This has been proven to be false. Ketones can cross the blood-brain barrier and support our brains when we don't have enough glucose. While some parts of the brain need glucose exclusively, we can produce the small amount we need via the protein we eat.

The breakdown of a keto diet is very simple. We aim for around 75% fat, 20% protein, and 5% carbs. The specific numbers in grams will differ, depending on your weight, but the math to figure it out is easy.

- **Fats.** For the average person on a 2000 calorie diet, we want around 110 grams of fat per day. For those working out and trying to build muscle, that number goes up as their caloric needs increase. The more active you are, the more energy your body needs; and therefore, you need more fat.
- **Protein.** On average, we want to stay between 0.6 and 0.9 grams of protein per pound of bodyweight for our daily intake. For example, if you weigh 175 pounds, you want to keep between 105 and 155 grams of protein per day.
- **Carbs.** For a 2000 calorie diet, we want the least amount of carbs reasonably possible. So, aiming for between 20 and 30 grams of carbs per day is best. That leaves us with enough room to keep a varied diet and account for the carbs we can't avoid in some foods.

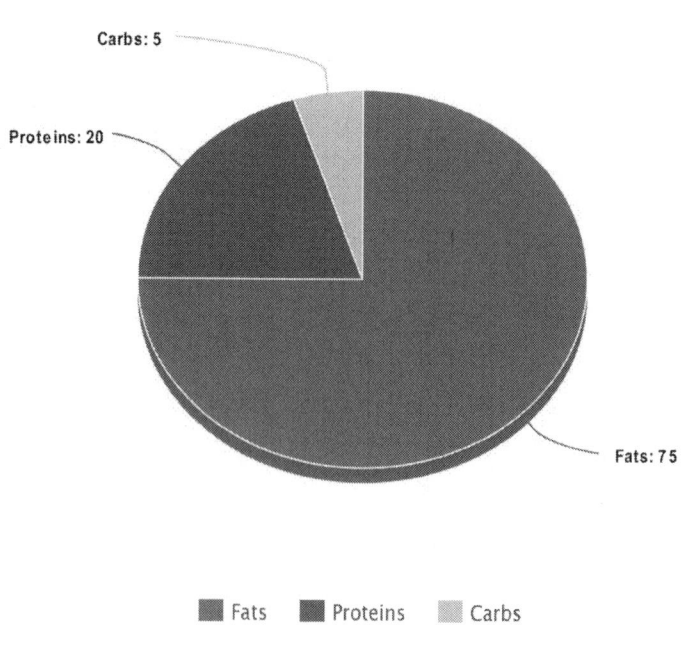

Chapter 2

Why Choose Keto?

Keto has a plethora of benefits for those willing to persevere and stick to the diet. Unlike so many other diets, keto has exemplary science behind it!

According to a study by experts at the Duke University Medical Center, keto diets are vastly superior to low-fat diets when it comes to weight loss and cardiovascular health (https://nutritionandmetabolism.biomedcentral.com/articles/10.1186/1743-7075-5-36). A study led by professors at the University of Cincinnati has shown that those who use a keto diet lose up to 2.2 times more weight than those on a low-fat diet (https://academic.oup.com/jcem/article/88/4/1617/2845298).

This incredible weight-loss is due to the fact our bodies are burning our fat reserves for energy, rather than the carbs we would usually ingest with each meal. Besides, keto diets are far more satiating than low-fat diets. This means we feel fuller after each meal and are less likely to snack during the day.

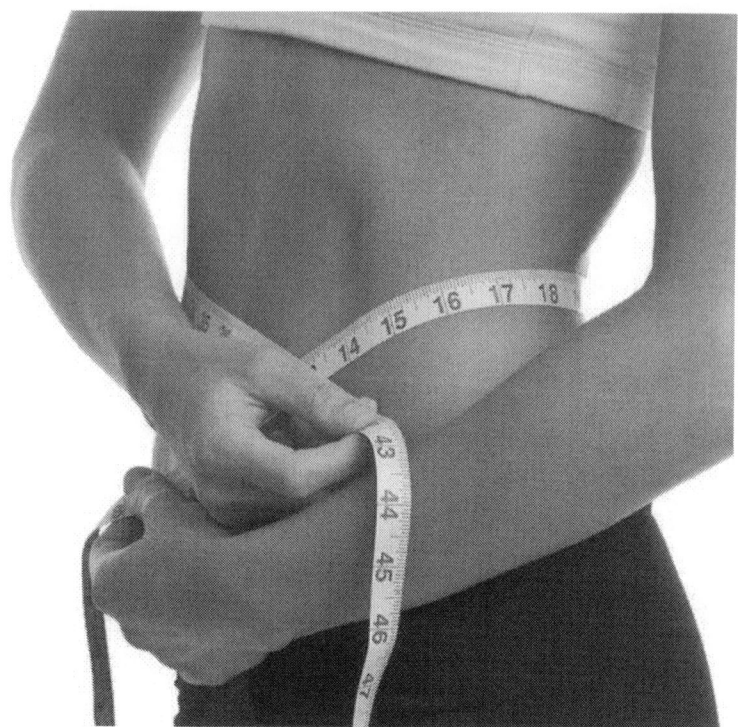

Coupled with weight loss, the keto diet has many other wide-ranging health benefits such as:

- **Improves insulin sensitivity.** Keto diets can lead to a 75% increase in insulin sensitivity, greatly helping those with type-2 diabetes. Test patients have been shown to need less medication over time as their bodies have adjusted to the keto diet.
- **Lowers chance of heart disease.** Reducing carbohydrate intake is a major factor in reducing heart disease risk factors like total cholesterol, triglycerides, and HDL cholesterol.
- **Acne.** The keto diet helps fight acne in the long term by lowering insulin and skin related hormone levels. Although initially, you may notice small breakouts while your body adjusts.
- **Overall skin health.** Besides helping with acne, the keto diet can help your skin in various other ways. The increase in

fat in your diet will help your skin nourish itself with more oil, causing it to glow and look healthier. Less sugar and starch in our diet also leads to fewer wrinkles and age lines. Too much sugar triggers a process called glycation, which produces molecules that weaken collagen.

- **Helps with Cancer therapy.** A clinical trial by members of the Albert Einstein College of Medicine in New York, found that ketosis has an effect on slowing the growth of cancer cells and helping bring about partial remission (https://www.sciencedirect.com/science/article/abs/pii/S0899900712001864?via%3Dihub). It is believed the absence of glucose helps starve cancer cells.
- **Boosts metabolism.** The increase in fat burning brought about by ketosis also leads to an increased metabolic rate. This is great for those of us who work busy days and warrants the extra energy.
- **Increases lean muscle mass.** Many athletes use the keto diet (or some form of it) to help increase their lean muscle mass. The lower carb and higher fat intake can result in an increase in muscle mass, strength, and energy over the course of the diet.
- **Reduction in seizures.** Keto diets have been proven to be incredibly effective in reducing the frequency of seizures in children and adolescents with epilepsy. Keto helps in this regard by modifying the genes related to energy metabolism in the brain, and this helps regulate the functions of neurons exposed to epilepsy.
- **Helps defeat sugar addiction.** Sugar addiction is a big issue many people who are looking to lose weight will face. It can be so hard to wean yourself off something that tastes so good and is available in so many foods. But keto meal plans are specially designed to avoid sugar and replace it with equally tasty, albeit far healthier alternatives.

As you can see, keto has a wide variety of amazing benefits. Every merit listed above has been confirmed by decades of meticulous research by doctors and dieticians worldwide. Many diets make lofty claims about what they can do for you, but keto is one of the few, which has the research to back it up properly.

Chapter 3

Where Do You Start?

After seeing how it works and the benefits, you may be left wondering, *where do I start?* In the comfort of your own home, of course! Keto isn't some super exercise focused diet, and we don't rely on group sessions or boot camps to help us lose weight. With keto, all we need is a simple diet change to get us started on our journey. Below I'll list and explain each change needed to get started on your keto diet:

- **Cut carbs.** The first and most important step to take towards the keto diet is cutting out carbs. I know it may sound very simple, even trivial, but it's a lot tougher than it seems for most of us. The majority of us will have bread, pasta, potatoes, rice, or something similar at least once a day, but in a keto diet that has to be avoided. As someone who loves pasta, this was incredibly hard for me, but I managed, and it paid off. For the average person, we want to stay below 50 grams of carbs per day; ideally, down to 20 grams per day.
- **Limit protein.** Now that we've cut out carbs, we need to replace them with the fatty foods that will power us when we reach ketosis. Many people make the mistake of replacing their carbs with protein, and this is an issue because excess protein can be converted into glucose. If we have excess proteins in our diet, we may find it harder to reach ketosis.
- **Avoid sugar.** Just because keto is a high-fat diet doesn't mean sugary foods are good for us. Glucose, fructose, and sucrose are all incredibly common in candy, soft drinks, and junk food that you come across. These sugars are the exact things that we are trying to remove by cutting carbs out of our diet. Aside from natural sugars, we should also refrain from sweeteners like xylitol, maltitol, aspartame, and

saccharin. These sweeteners have similar net carbs to pure table sugar and should be avoided all the same.
- **Keep your vegetables above ground!** Vegetables are an important part of keto, but we want to include only above-ground vegetables in our meals. Root vegetables are high in starch and sugars, while the vast majority of green vegetables are light on carbs. Some of the best vegetables for keto include lettuce, spinach, asparagus, avocado, cauliflower, cucumber, and tomato.

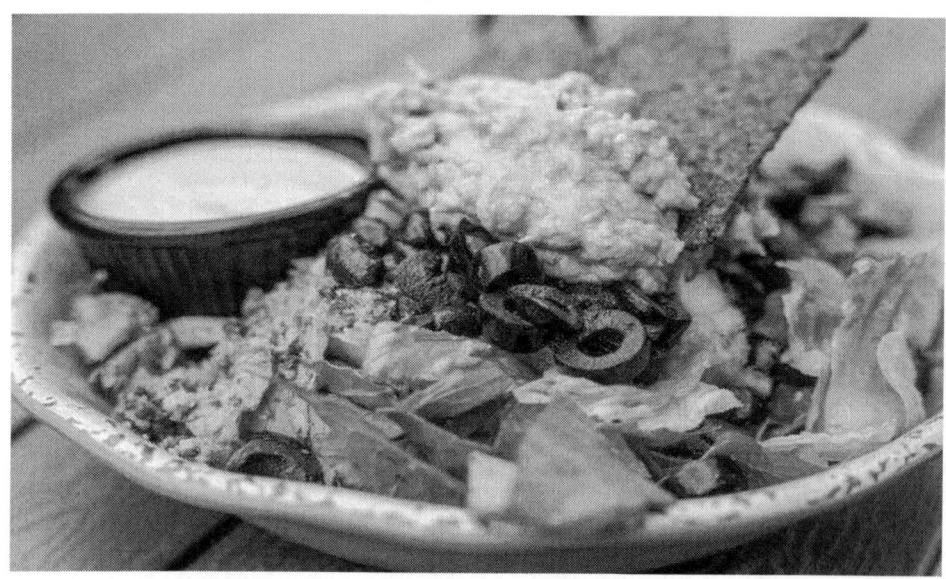

- **Be careful with what you drink.** Many people overlook their drinks, while dieting but we won't make that same mistake. In keto, the drinks you have during the day can make or break your path to ketosis. Luckily, we have plenty of healthy options when it comes to refreshments. We've all been taught since we were children that you should always drink plenty of water, and there isn't any reason not to. Put slices of lemon or lime into your glass, and there you have a delicious drink with *zero* carbs. Tea and coffee are fantastic too, but avoid using any of the sugars or sweeteners mentioned above, and be careful using too much milk. Diet soft drinks can be fine as well, be careful to read the ingredients. Many diet drinks may have sweeteners which are still carb heavy. Lastly, alcohol is actually very light on carbs. Wine and pure spirits are all fine to drink on a keto diet.

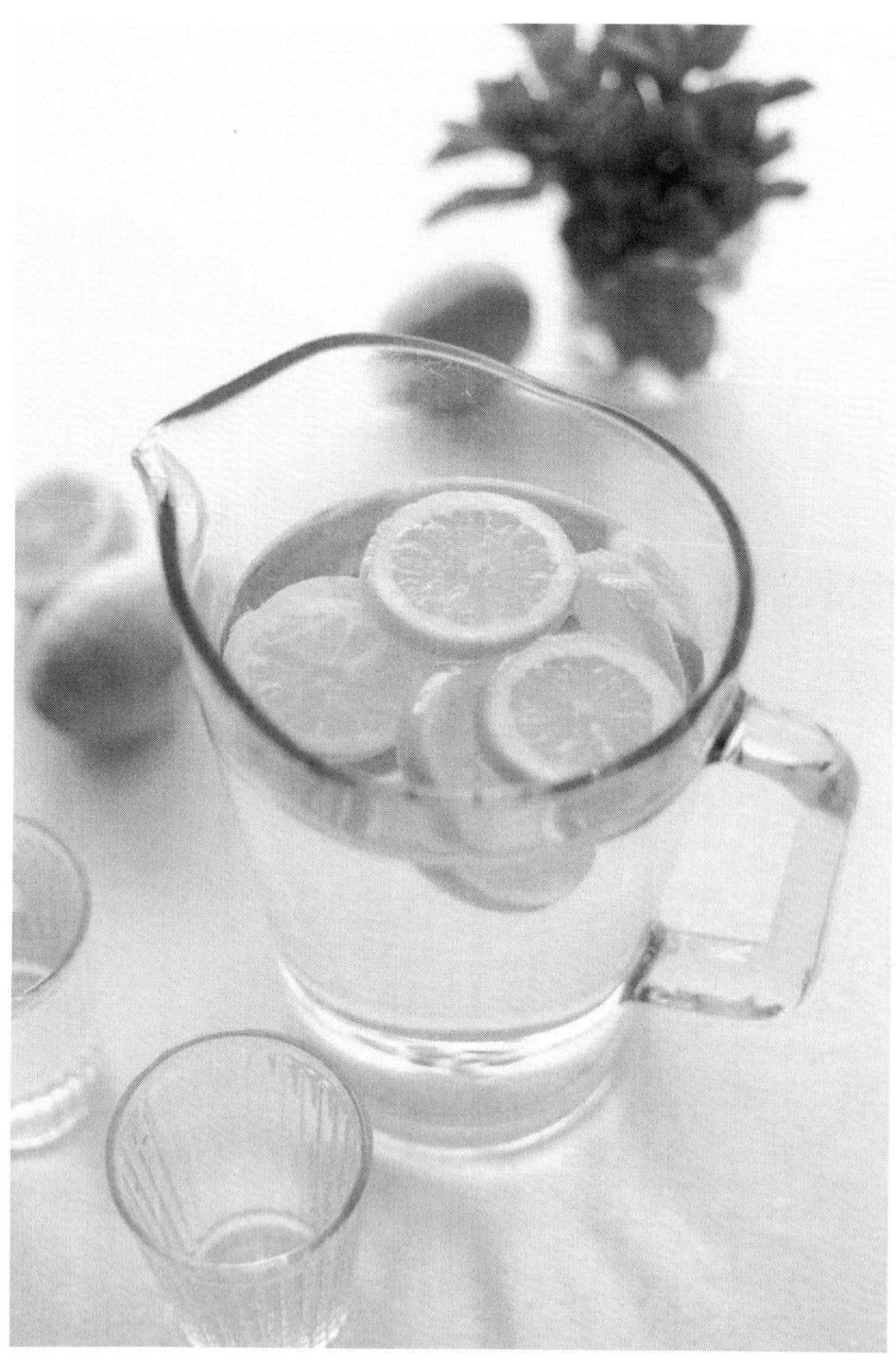

- **Increase healthy fats!** As we've already stated, the keto diet is high-fat. Because we've been taught to avoid fat for so many years, it is often hard to wrap our heads around needing more than 60% fat in our daily diet. Luckily there are easy and healthy ways of increasing your fat intake. One tasty and easy to find a source of healthy fats is via fish. Salmon, mackerel, herring, and sardines are great examples of fatty fish, all of which are easy to source and make for tasty meals. Another fantastic source of fats is oil. Coconut, avocado, and olive oil are healthy choices of oil, which we can use for cooking meals and garnishing vegetables. Lastly, animal products are also a great way of obtaining your healthy fats quota for the day. Eggs, cheese, butter, and cream can make for perfect snacks throughout the day, especially when partnered with low carb nuts such as pecans, macadamias, and brazil nuts.

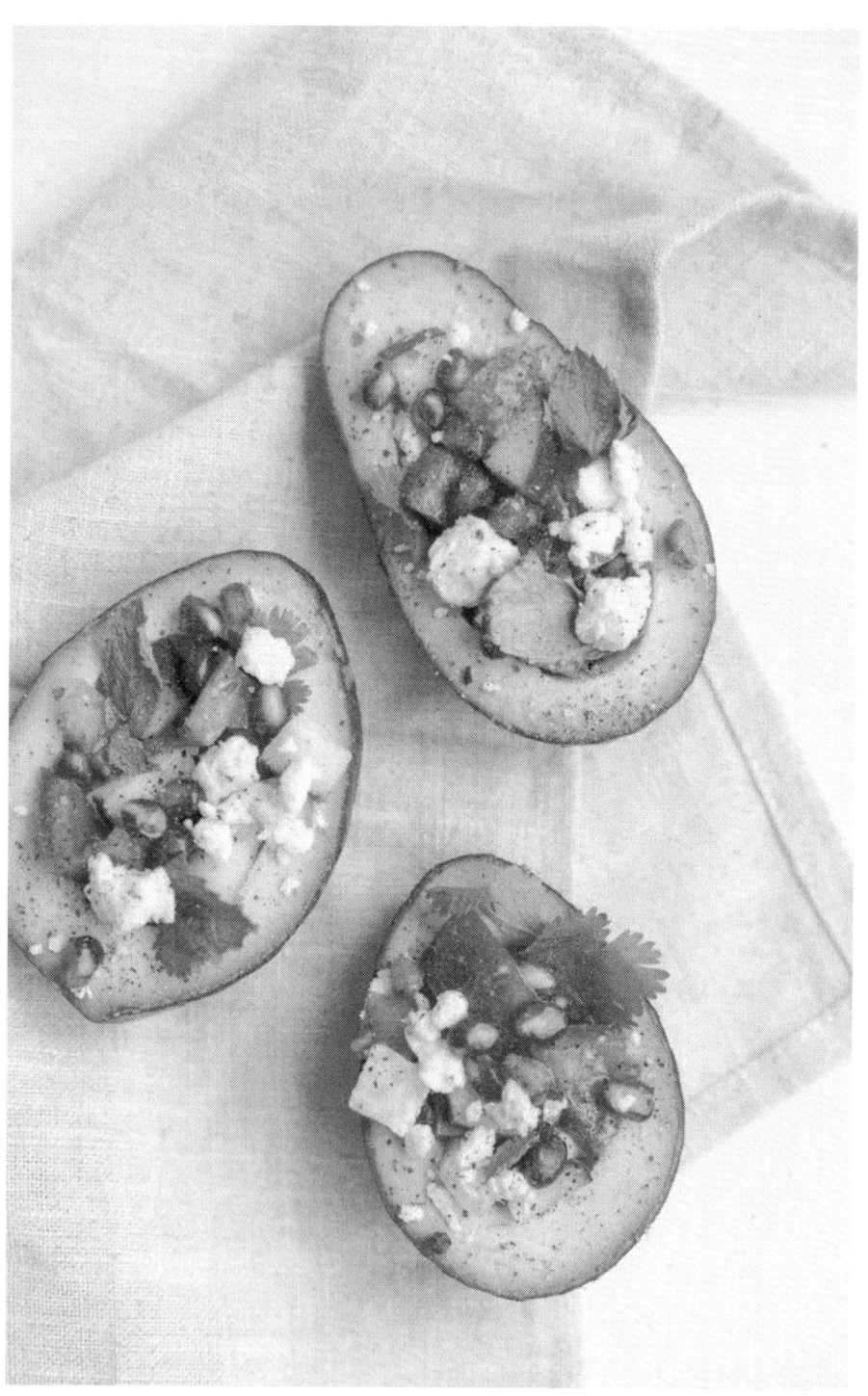

- **Use a calorie counter.** Even if you're following a meticulous meal plan, keep a calorie counter with you. We must hold ourselves to the requirements of our keto diet. Having an app or notepad that allows us to track our meals will help us learn more about our diet and how to better reach our goals.

I know new diets can be hard in the beginning, but the beauty about keto is that every change you need to make is easily achievable. It's a series of small easy steps that lead to an incredible end result. Take your time to work these changes into your daily life, and don't rush. Keto done at your own pace is the best kind of keto!

Chapter 4

The Secret Ingredient

Now that you know how keto works and how to get started, I'm going to share with you the (not so) secret keys to a successful diet: a calorie deficit and moderate exercise! As obvious as that may sound, far too many people overlook these two simple points.

Calories

In high-fat diets like keto, sometimes we feel a bit too indulgent with what we eat, it's a fatty diet after all, right? Regardless of the composition of our meals, it's still a diet, which means to have any hope of losing weight; we need to eat fewer calories than our body burns. Your guide or meal plan may already have a calculated deficit for you, but if you're forging your own path and want to figure out what deficit is good for you, then it is pretty easy to figure out. You need to understand two things before you figure out your deficit, how many calories do I need to be healthy? And how fast do I want to lose weight?

Let's start with "how many calories do I need to be healthy?" The answer to this question depends on your age, gender, and level of activity, but to make things easy, I've included graphs below. As you age, your caloric needs increase and decrease, our peak is hit between the ages of 15 and 25 where our bodies do most of their growing. As you get older, your body stops growing, and your metabolism slows, so you need fewer calories to operate. By the time you hit your late 50s, your required daily intake will be nearly 500 calories less than earlier in your life. This is important to note that many people don't adjust their diets to match their caloric needs as they age, and it has led to high levels of obesity in the older population of many first world countries.

The graphs below show the daily minimum required calorie intake for moderately active men and women of various age groups. If you're sedentary (desk job, disabled, bedridden), you may need up to 200 calories less than the average moderately active adult. Conversely, if you're an active person who regularly goes to the gym or takes part in sports, you may need up to 400 calories more.

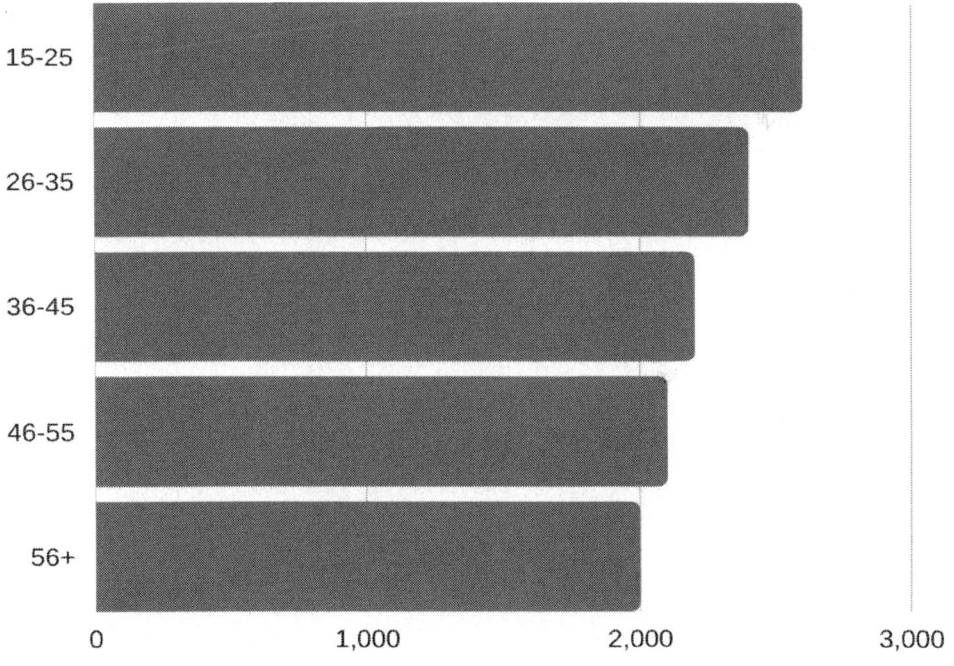

Minimum Healthy Calorie Intake for Moderately Active Men

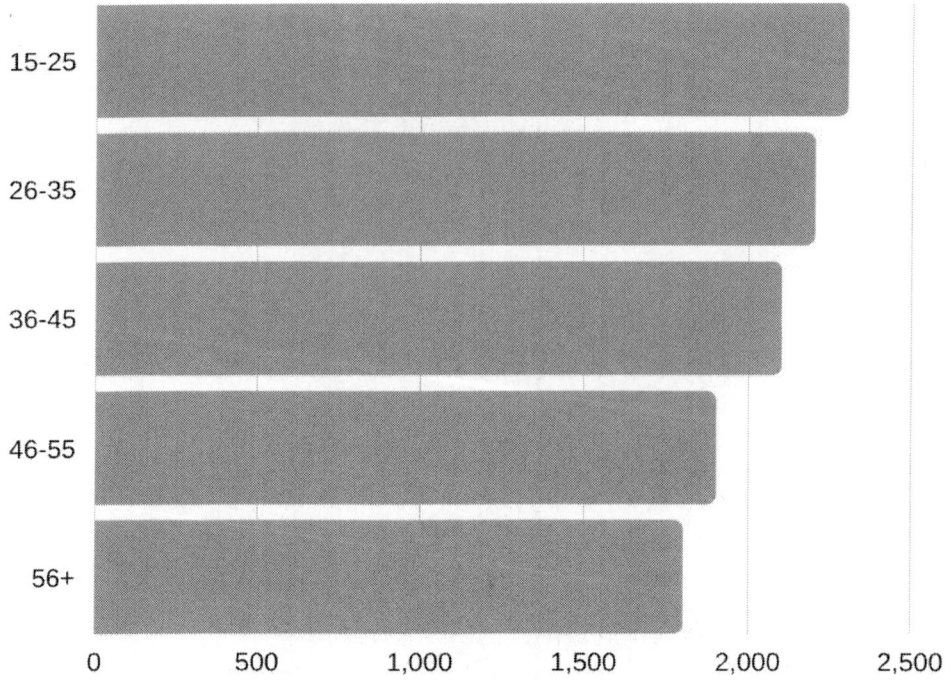

Minimum Healthy Calorie Intake for Moderately Active Women

Exercise

The second half of our secret ingredient is exercise. As people, we tend to dread exercise; it's sweaty and uncomfortable, tiring, and sometimes time-consuming, but absolutely necessary. Luckily, unlike many other diets, keto doesn't expect a rigorous exercise regime from you. Moderate activity is all that is needed to succeed with keto. It may sound too good to be true, but the logic behind it is fairly simple.

With a keto diet, the majority of our fat burning is done by our organs to produce energy, unlike other diets that rely on our muscles burning fat during exercise. Although, this doesn't mean that you can get away with doing no exercise. For the best results in weight-loss and general health, it's always best to stay active.

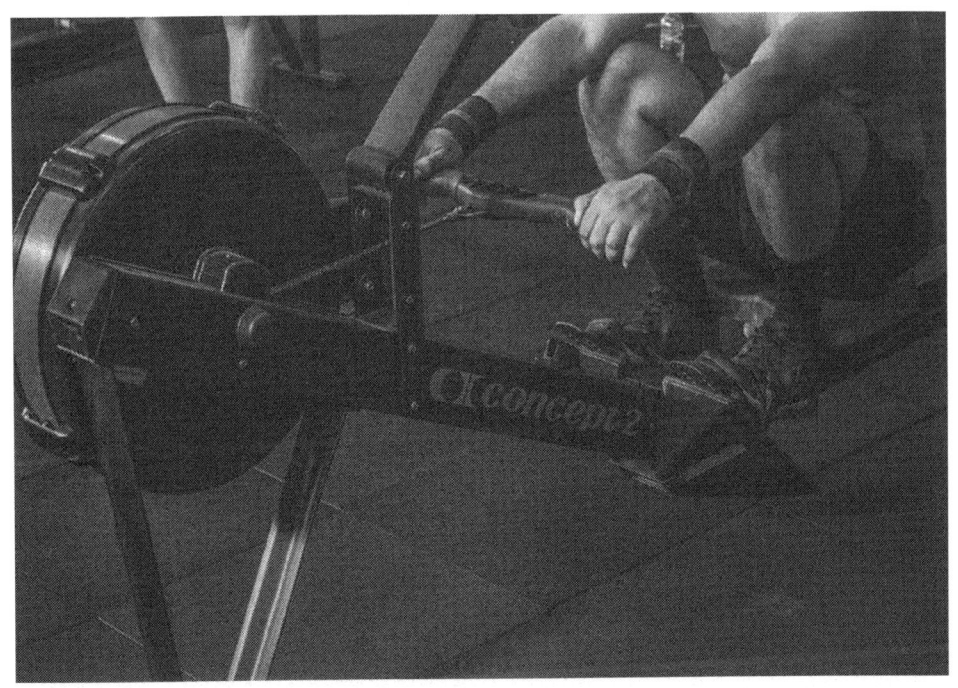

The keto diet doesn't restrict you in any way regarding workouts; you can still do them all. But, it has been shown that specific exercises benefit your body more on a keto diet than normally would in any other diet. These exercises tend to be focused on endurance and cardio. Rowing, biking, jogging, and yoga, particularly, all benefit massively from the steady, slow-burning energy that a keto diet gives you. Exercises like weight lifting and sprinting, although good for you, may not offer the same results on a keto diet as they normally would. When it comes to building bulk muscle mass, the keto diet isn't ideal as you need a surplus of protein.

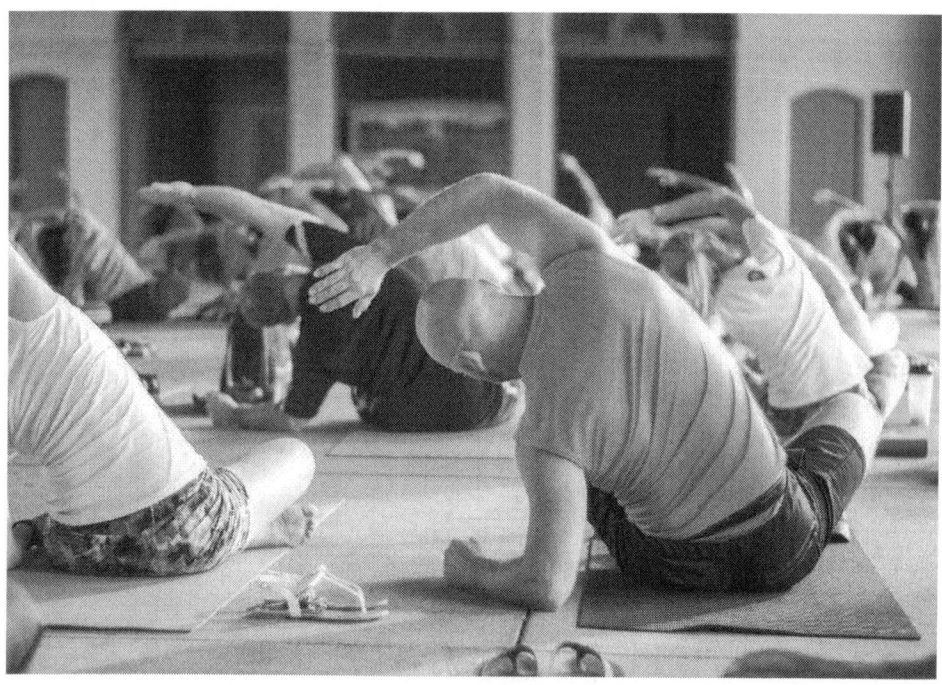

Cardio exercises primarily work on burning fat for energy, considering this is the core concept of a keto diet we can use this to incredible effect. Jogging, for example, is one of the best all-round exercises you can do. Not only does it work out multiple parts of your body, but it increases your endurance, agility, and balance.

When you jog, your heart rate increases, your blood pumps faster, and your breathing is harder. This increase in activity among your muscles and major organs means your body needs to supply more energy to keep up. This typically means that your body starts burning its fat reserves to sustain this sudden increase in activity. For those on the keto diet, this is great, since your body is already burning fat passively for energy, so any cardio exercise speeds up the process. This same logic applies to any form of endurance exercise, so keto and cardio go hand-in-hand.

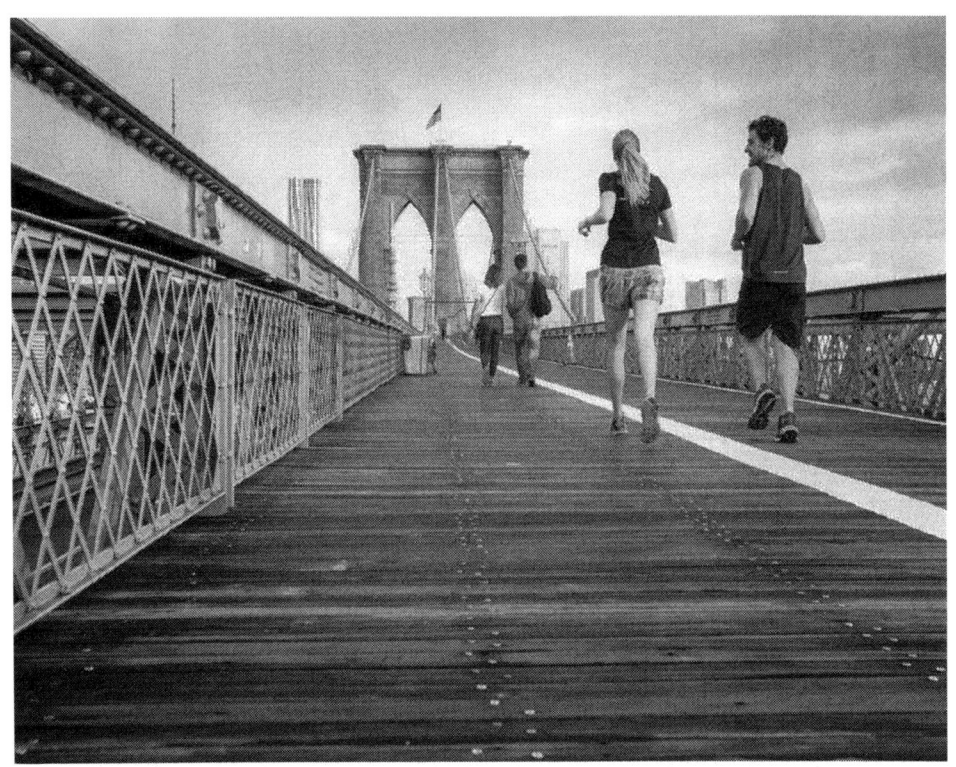

Chapter 5

THE 30-Day KETO DIET MEAL PLAN TO LET YOU SUCCEED!

Here's first option for lunch if you want more variety. The second option for lunch is to use the dinner leftovers for lunch, so this will save time.

Day 1:

Breakfast – Vegetable Scrambled Eggs

Lunch – Lettuce and Avocado Sandwiches

Dinner – Bacon-Wrapped Salmon

Day 2:

Breakfast – Chicken and Bacon Pancake

Lunch – Meat Muffin

Dinner – Bacon-Wrapped Salmon

Day 3:

Breakfast – Cheesy Vegetable Frittata

Lunch – Berries in Yogurt Cream

Dinner – Herbed Steaks

Day 4:

Breakfast – Sausage and Fried Eggs

Lunch – Avocado and Salmon

Dinner – Pumpkin Soup

Day 5:

Breakfast – Mozzarella and Garlic Waffles

Lunch – Cheesy Deviled Eggs with Avocado

Dinner – Shrimp and Bacon

Day 6:

Breakfast – Peanut Butter Oatmeal

Lunch – Lettuce Wraps

Dinner – Chili

Day 7:

Breakfast – Cheese Omelet

Lunch – Cider Chicken Thighs

Dinner – Teriyaki Chicken

Day 8:

Breakfast – Egg Muffin

Lunch – Cheese Muffin

Dinner – Roasted Cauliflower Steaks

Day 9:

Breakfast – Breakfast Tuna Wrap

Lunch – Spinach Stuffed Zucchini

Dinner – Chicken and Coconut Curry

Day 10:

Breakfast – Beef and Spinach Frittata

Lunch – Cheesy Cauliflower Soup

Dinner – Tuna and Spinach Salad

Day 11:

Breakfast – Pumpkin Spiced Hemp Porridge

Lunch – Tuna Egg Boats

Dinner – Beef and Broccoli

Day 12:

Breakfast – Breakfast Patties

Lunch – Ranch Deviled Eggs

Dinner – Chicken Nuggets

Day 13:

Breakfast – Eggs in Clouds

Lunch – Broccoli and Bacon Salad

Dinner – Chicken Nuggets

Day 14:

Breakfast – Jalapeno Waffle

Lunch – Paprika Chicken

Dinner – Coconut Crusted Fish

Day 15:

Breakfast – Bacon and Egg Breakfast Muffin

Lunch – Garlic Zoodles

Dinner – Pork Chops with Mushrooms

Day 16:

Breakfast – Bagel

Lunch – Sweet and Spicy Brussel Sprouts

Dinner – Cheesy Chicken Stuffed Bell Pepper

Day 17:

Breakfast – Breakfast Vanilla Pudding

Lunch – Salmon Patties

Dinner – Buttery Salmon

Day 18:

Breakfast – Cheesy Avocado Egg Boat

Lunch – Stuffed Zucchini Boats

Dinner – Cheddar Chicken

Day 19:

Breakfast – Beef Omelet Wrap

Lunch – Caprese Salad

Dinner – Meatloaf

Day 20:

Breakfast – Cream Cheese Pancake

Lunch – Egg and Spinach Salad with Bacon

Dinner – Red Curry Glazed Fish

Day 21:

Breakfast – Spinach Egg Muffin

Lunch – Lime and Garlic Chicken Thighs

Dinner – Chicken Salad

Day 22:

Breakfast – Boiled Eggs and Avocado Plate

Lunch – Cheesy Zoodles

Dinner – Bacon Wrapped Chicken

Day 23:

Breakfast – Cauliflower Hash Browns

Lunch – Tuna Cakes

Dinner – Beef and Spinach Sliders

Day 24:

Breakfast – Waffles with Poached Eggs

Lunch – Pork and Egg Cup

Dinner – Pulled Chicken

Day 25:

Breakfast – Cinnamon Muffin

Lunch – Taco Radish Wedges

Dinner – Cocoa Rubbed Pork

Day 26:

Breakfast – Porridge

Lunch – Spinach Salad with Feta Dressing

Dinner – Basil Stuffed Chicken

Day 27:

Breakfast – Bacon and Egg Cup

Lunch – Asparagus Sauté with Bacon

Dinner – Salmon with Green Beans

Day 28:

Breakfast – Cheesy Garlic Bacon Knots

Lunch – Tuna Salad

Dinner – Cream of Asparagus Soup

Day 29:

Breakfast – Bell Pepper Eggs

Lunch – Marinara Deviled Egg

Dinner – Creamy Chicken Soup

Day 30:

Breakfast – Breakfast Egg Salad

Lunch – Asparagus and Tomato Salad

Dinner – Cheesy Kale Patties

BREAKFAST

Vegetable Scrambled Eggs

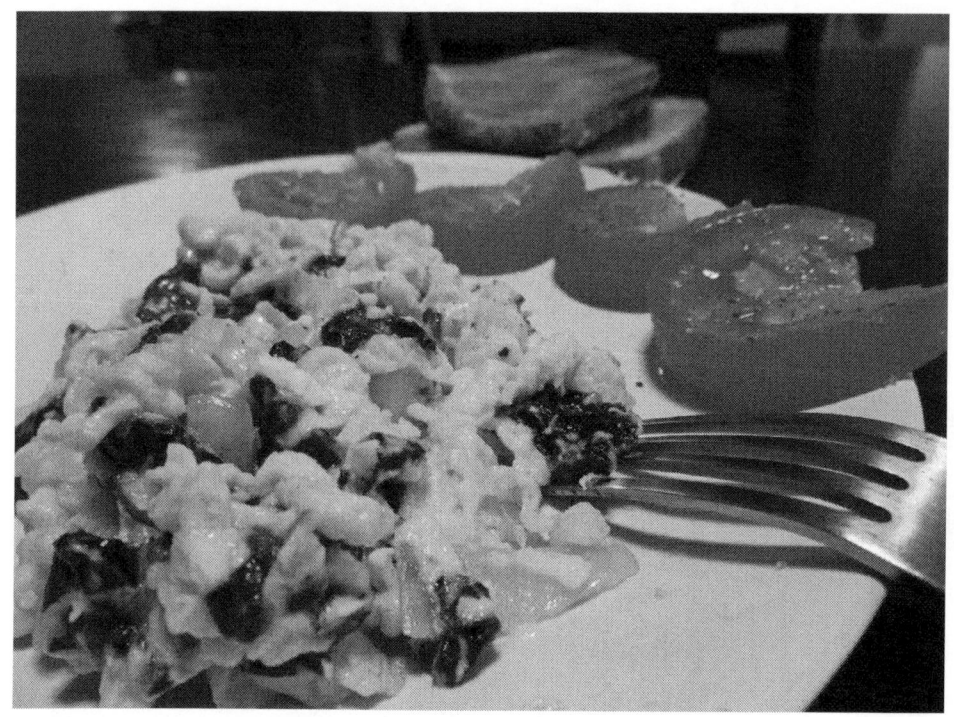

Nutrition Facts Per Serving

Calories	Fats	Proteins	Carbohydrates
156	13.3	7.7	0.8

Ingredients

Serves	1	2	3	4	5	6	7	8
Kale, chopped, cup	¼	½	¾	1	1 ¼	1 ½	1 ¾	2
Garlic powder, teaspoon	1/16	1/8	¼	1/3	½	2/3	¾	1
Egg, at room temperature	1	2	3	4	5	6	7	8
Avocado oil, tablespoon	½	1	1 ½	2	2 ½	3	3 ½	4
Cheddar cheese, grated, full-fat, tablespoon	½	1	1 ½	2	2 ½	3	3 ½	4
Salt, teaspoon	1/8	¼	1/3	½	2/3	¾	1	1 1/8

Instructions

1. Place the oil in a medium-sized skillet pan over medium heat. Upon hot, add the kale.
2. Season the kale with salt and garlic powder, stir until mixed, and then cook for 1 minute until the kale wilts.
3. Meanwhile, crack the egg in a bowl and then whisk until blended.
4. After 1 minute, pour the egg over the kale, stir until mixed, and then cook for 1 to 2 minutes until the eggs have scrambled.
5. When done, sprinkle the cheese over eggs, remove the pan from heat, and let the scrambled eggs rest for 1 minute.
6. Serve immediately.

Egg Muffin

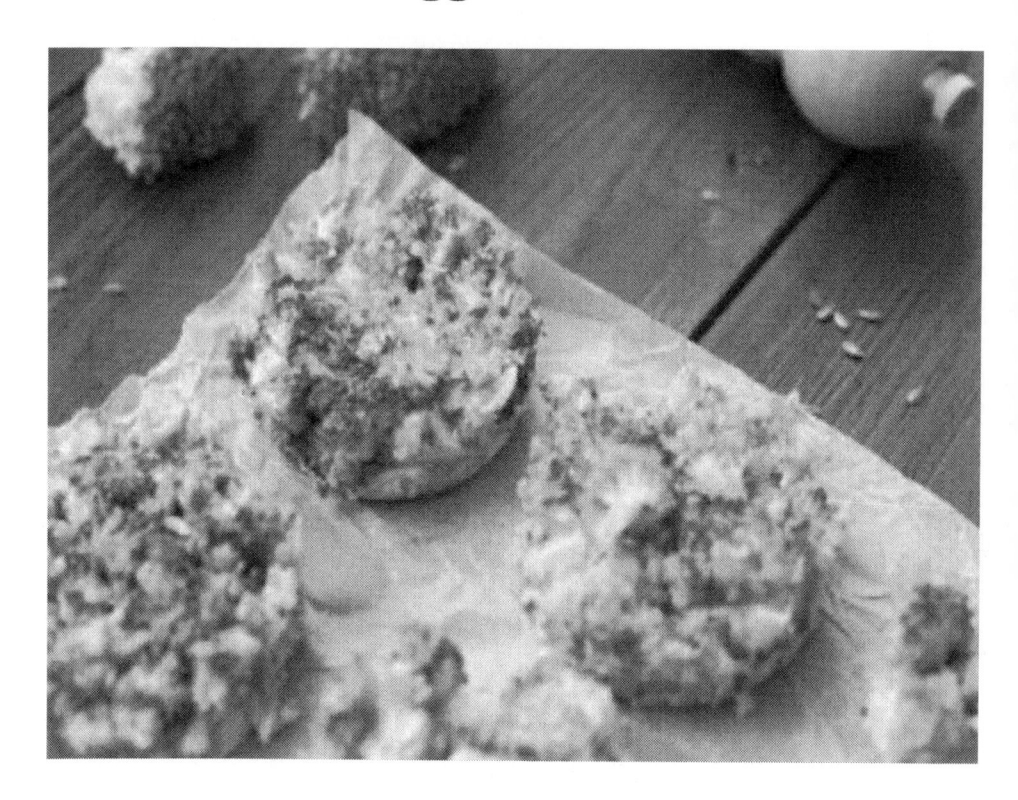

Nutrition Facts Per Serving

Calories	Fats	Proteins	Carbohydrates
110.1	7.7	8.8	1.4

Ingredients

Serves	1	2	3	4	5	6	7	8
Broccoli florets, tablespoon	2	4	6	8	10	12	14	16
Cheddar cheese, grated, full-fat, tablespoon	1	2	3	4	5	6	7	8
Dried thyme, teaspoon	1/16	1/8	1/4	1/3	½	2/3	¾	1
Egg, at room temperature	1	2	3	4	5	6	7	8
Salt, by taste	1/8	1/4	1/3	½	2/3	¾	1	1 1/8
Black pepper, by taste	1/8	1/4	1/3	½	2/3	¾	1	1 1/8

Instructions

1. Turn on the oven, set it 400 degrees F, and let it preheat.
2. In the meantime, place the florets in a small heatproof bowl, cover it with plastic wrap, poke some holes in it, and then microwave for 30 to 60 seconds until florets have steamed.
3. Take a silicone muffin cup, spray it with avocado oil, and then drain broccoli and transfer it into the prepared muffin cup.
4. Crack the egg in a small bowl, add salt, black pepper, and thyme, and then whisk until blended.
5. Top the broccoli with cheese, pour in the blended egg, and then bake for 8 to 10 minutes until firm and the top turn golden brown.
6. Serve right away.

Sausage and Fried Eggs

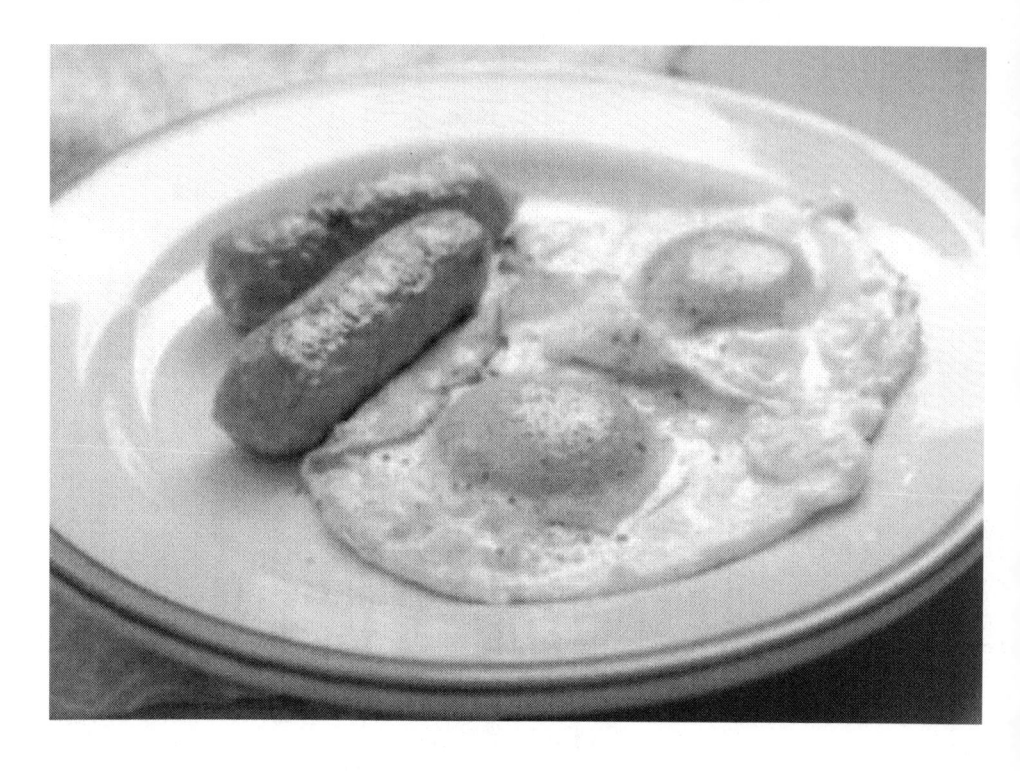

Nutrition Facts Per Serving

Calories	Fats	Proteins	Carbohydrates
448	32.9	33.6	4.5

Ingredients

Serves	1	2	3	4	5	6	7	8
Sausage links	2	4	6	8	10	12	14	16
Egg	1	2	3	4	5	6	7	8
Avocado oil, tablespoon	2	4	6	8	10	12	14	16
Salt, by taste								
Black pepper, by taste								

Instructions

1. Place the oil in a medium skillet pan over medium heat and let it warm.
2. Place the sausages in it and then cook them for 3 to 4 minutes per side until nicely browned and cooked.
3. Push the cooked sausages to one side of the pan, add the oil on the other side of the pan, and let it heat.
4. Then crack the egg on the other side of the pan and fry it for 3 to 4 minutes until cooked to the desired level.
5. Transfer the sausages and the fried egg to a plate, sprinkle salt and black pepper over them, and then serve.

Boiled Eggs and Avocado Plate

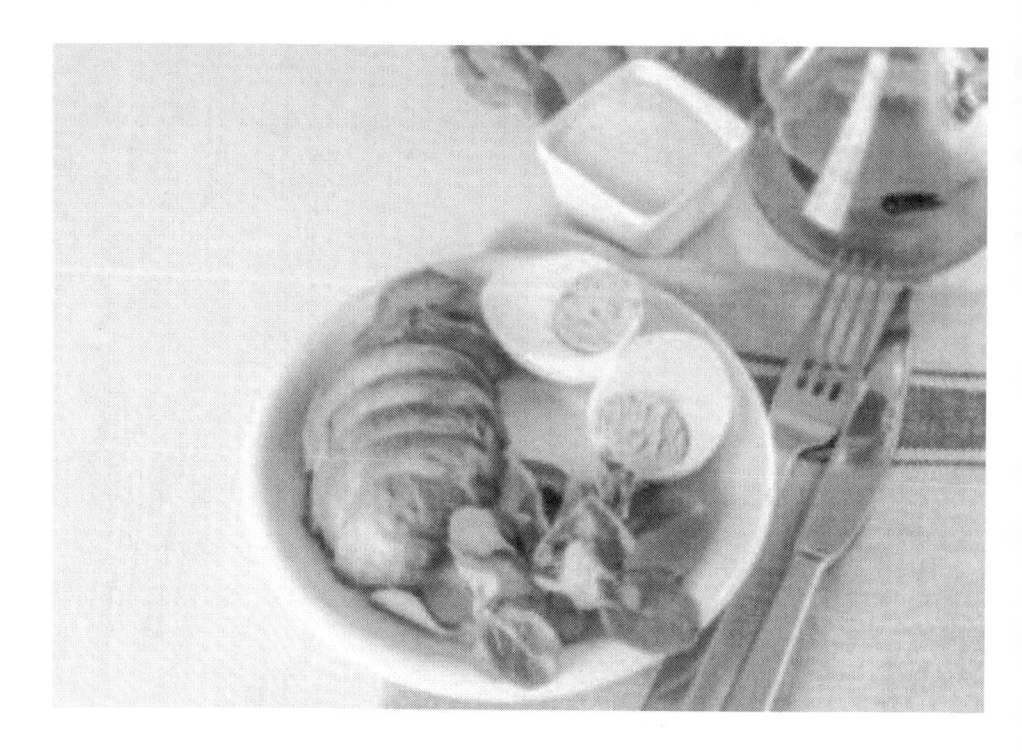

Nutrition Facts Per Serving

Calories	Fats	Proteins	Carbohydrates
389	33.7	17.5	3.9

Ingredients

Serves	1	2	3	4	5	6	7	8
Egg	2	4	6	8	10	12	14	16
Avocado, peeled, pitted, flesh sliced	½	1	1 ½	2	2 ½	3	3 ½	4
Avocado oil, tablespoon	1	2	3	4	5	6	7	8
Salt, by taste								
Black pepper, by taste								

Instructions

1. Fill a small pot with water until half full, place it over medium heat, and then bring it to boil.
2. Then carefully lower the eggs into the pot and boil it for 5 to 10 minutes until cooked to the desired level, for soft-boiled cook it for 5 minutes, for medium-boiled cook it for 8 minutes, and for hard-boiled cook it for 10 minutes.
3. When done, transfer the eggs to a bowl filled with chilled water and let it rest for 5 minutes until cooled enough to be peeled.
4. Peel the eggs, cut them into slices, and place onto a plate.
5. Add the avocado slices, sprinkle salt and black pepper over the boiled eggs and avocado slices, drizzle with oil, and then serve.

Breakfast Patties

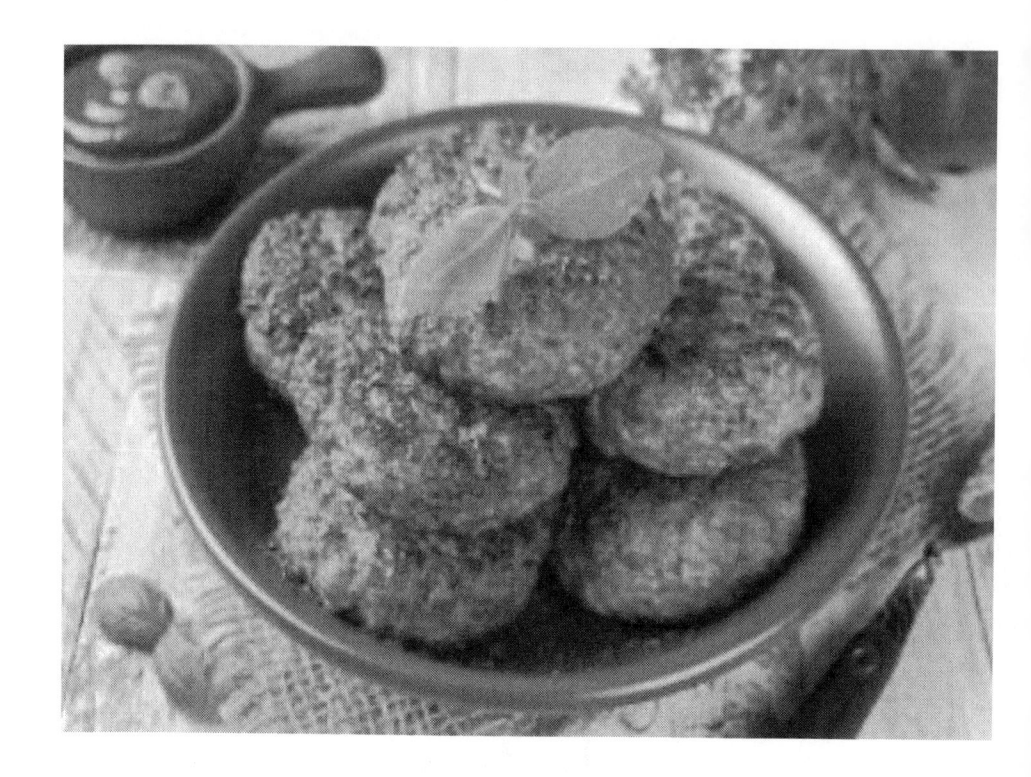

Nutrition Facts Per Serving

Calories	Fats	Proteins	Carbohydrates
588	37.2	63.2	0

Ingredients

Serves	1	2	3	4	5	6	7	8
Ground beef, pound	½	1	1 ½	2	2 ½	3	3 ½	4
Garlic powder	½	1	1 ½	2	2 ½	3	3 ½	4
Smoked paprika	½	1	1 ½	2	2 ½	3	3 ½	4
Avocado oil, tablespoon	2	4	6	8	10	12	14	16
Salt, teaspoon	½	1	1 ½	2	2 ½	3	3 ½	4
Black pepper, teaspoon	¼	½	¾	1	1 ¼	1 ½	1 ¾	2

Instructions

1. Place the beef in a medium bowl, add garlic powder, paprika, salt, and black pepper, stir until mixed, and then shape the mixture into two patties.
2. Place the oil in a medium frying pan, place it over medium heat and let it heat.
3. Arrange the prepared patties in it and then cook for 4 to 6 minutes per side until golden brown and thoroughly cooked.
4. Serve right away.

Bacon and Egg Breakfast Muffin

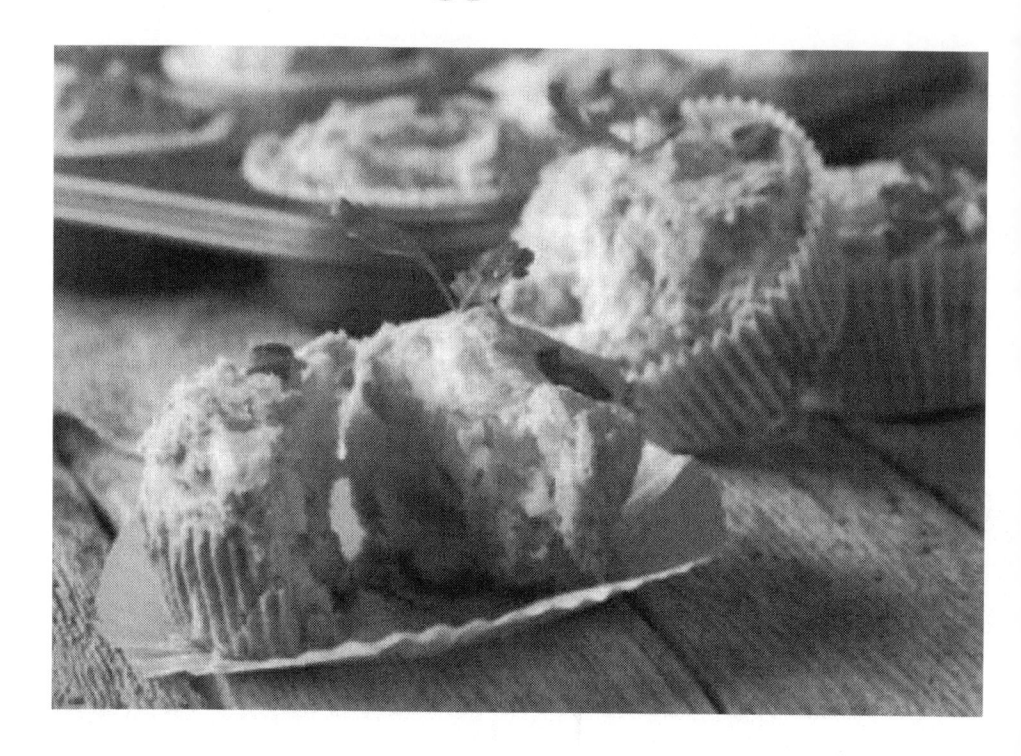

Nutrition Facts Per Serving

Calories	Fats	Proteins	Carbohydrates
412	36.2	20.6	1

Ingredients

Serves	1	2	3	4	5	6	7	8
Bacon slices	1	2	3	4	5	6	7	8
Chopped green onion, tablespoon	¼	½	¾	1	1¼	1½	1¾	2
Chopped parsley, tablespoon	¼	½	¾	1	1¼	1½	1¾	2
Egg, at room temperature	1	2	3	4	5	6	7	8
Heavy cream, full-fat, tablespoon	½	1	1 ½	2	2 ½	3	3 ½	4

Instructions

1. Switch on the oven, then set it to 375 degrees F, and let it preheat.
2. In the meantime, place a frying pan over medium heat and when hot, place bacon slice and cook it for 2 to 3 minutes per side until crisp and cooked.
3. Transfer the bacon to a cutting board, let it cool for 5 minutes, and then chop it.
4. Crack the egg in a small bowl, whisk it until blended and then stir in onion, parsley, bacon, and cream until combined.
5. Take a silicone muffin cups, grease it with avocado spray, fill with bacon mixture, and then bake for 8 to 12 minutes until firm and the top have turned golden brown.
6. Serve immediately.

Spinach Egg Muffin

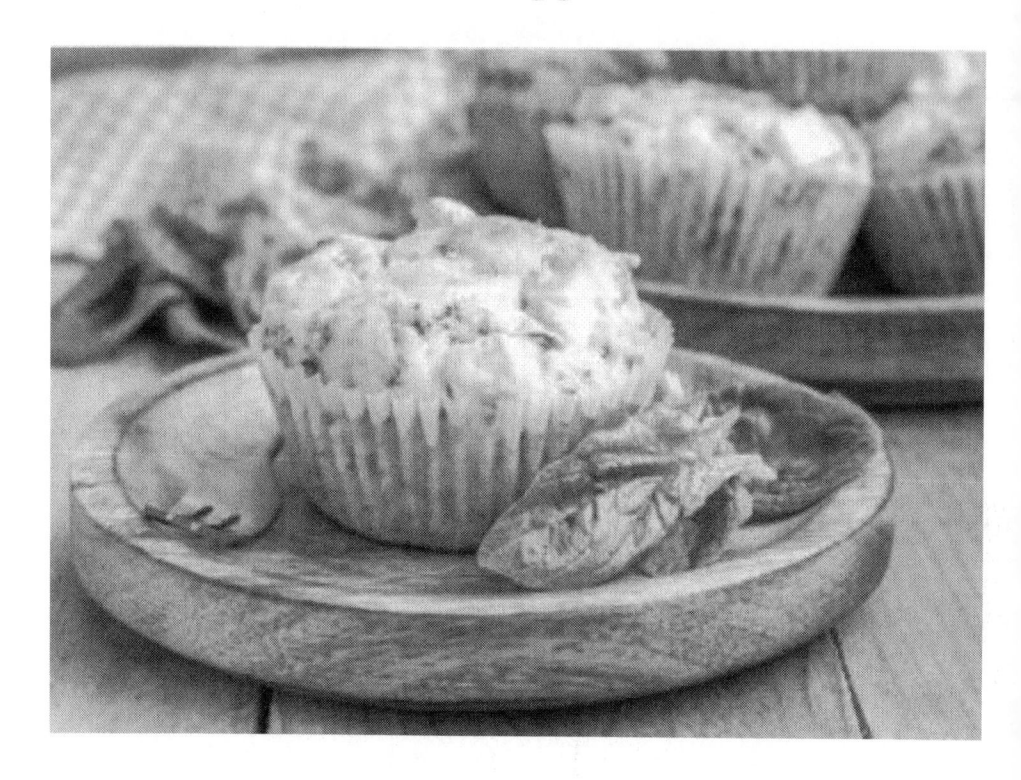

Nutrition Facts Per Serving

Calories	Fats	Proteins	Carbohydrates
132	8.8	10.9	2.3

Ingredients

Serves	1	2	3	4	5	6	7	8
Chopped spinach, fresh, cup	¼	½	¾	1	1¼	1½	1¾	2
Dried basil, teaspoon	1/8	1/4	1/3	½	2/3	¾	1	1 1/8
Egg, at room temperature	1	2	3	4	5	6	7	8
Parmesan cheese, grated, full-fat, tablespoon	1	2	3	4	5	6	7	8
Salt, teaspoon	1/16	1/8	1/4	1/3	½	2/3	¾	1
Black pepper, teaspoon	1/16	1/8	1/4	1/3	½	2/3	¾	1

Instructions

1. Switch on the oven, then set it to 400 degrees F, and let it preheat.
2. In the meantime, crack the egg in a small bowl, add basil, salt, and black pepper and then whisk until blended.
3. Add the spinach and cheese, and then stir until mixed.
4. Take a silicone muffin cup, grease it with avocado spray, fill with spinach batter, and then bake for 8 to 10 minutes until firm and the top turn golden brown.
5. Serve immediately.

Cheese Omelet

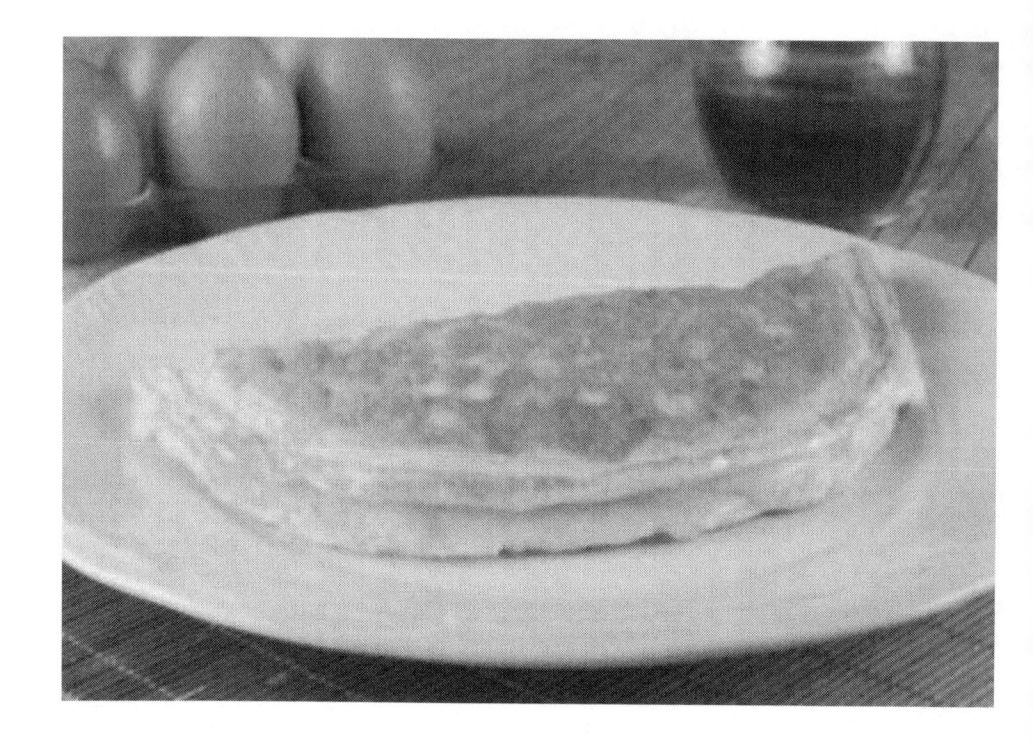

Nutrition Facts Per Serving

Calories	Fats	Proteins	Carbohydrates
224	19.9	10.1	1.1

Ingredients

Serves	1	2	3	4	5	6	7	8
Butter, unsalted, tablespoon	1	2	3	4	5	6	7	8
Egg	1	2	3	4	5	6	7	8
Mozzarella cheese, grated, full-fat	2	4	6	8	10	12	14	16
Salt, by taste								
Black pepper, by taste								

Instructions

1. Crack the egg in a small bowl, add salt, black pepper, and half of the cheese, and then whisk until blended.
2. Place the butter in a medium frying pan over medium-low heat, and when it melts, pour in the egg, and then spread it evenly.
3. Cook for 2 minutes until set, switch heat to medium, sprinkle remaining cheese over the egg, and then turn one half over other.
4. Slide the omelet to the plate and then serve.

Breakfast Egg Salad

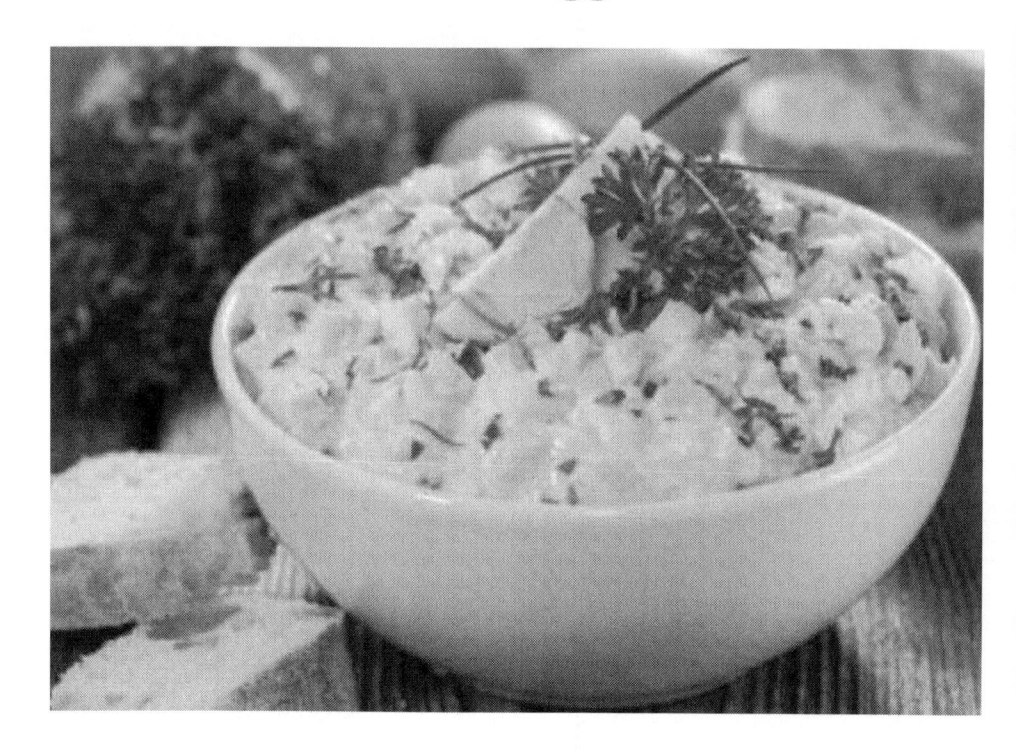

Nutrition Facts Per Serving

Calories	Fats	Proteins	Carbohydrates
356	30.5	19.6	0.9

Ingredients

Serves	1	2	3	4	5	6	7	8
Mayonnaise, tablespoons	2	4	6	8	10	12	14	16
Lemon juice, teaspoon	1	2	3	4	5	6	7	8
Egg, hard boiled	2	4	6	8	10	12	14	16
Slices of bacon	2	4	6	8	10	12	14	16
Salt, by taste								
Black pepper, by taste								

Instructions

1. Place a frying pan over medium heat and when hot, add the bacon slice, and cook it for 2 to 3 minutes per side until crisp and cooked.
2. Transfer the bacon to a cutting board, let it cool for 5 minutes, and then chop it.
3. Fill a small pot with water until half full, place it over medium heat and then bring it to boil.
4. Then carefully lower the eggs into the pot and boil it for 10 minutes until hard-boiled.
5. When done, transfer the eggs to a bowl filled with chilled water, let them rest for 5 minutes until cooled enough to be peeled, then peel the eggs, and dice them.
6. Add diced eggs to a bowl, stir in mayonnaise, salt, black pepper, and lemon juice, and then stir mix combined.
7. Top the salad with bacon and then serve.

Bacon and Egg Cup

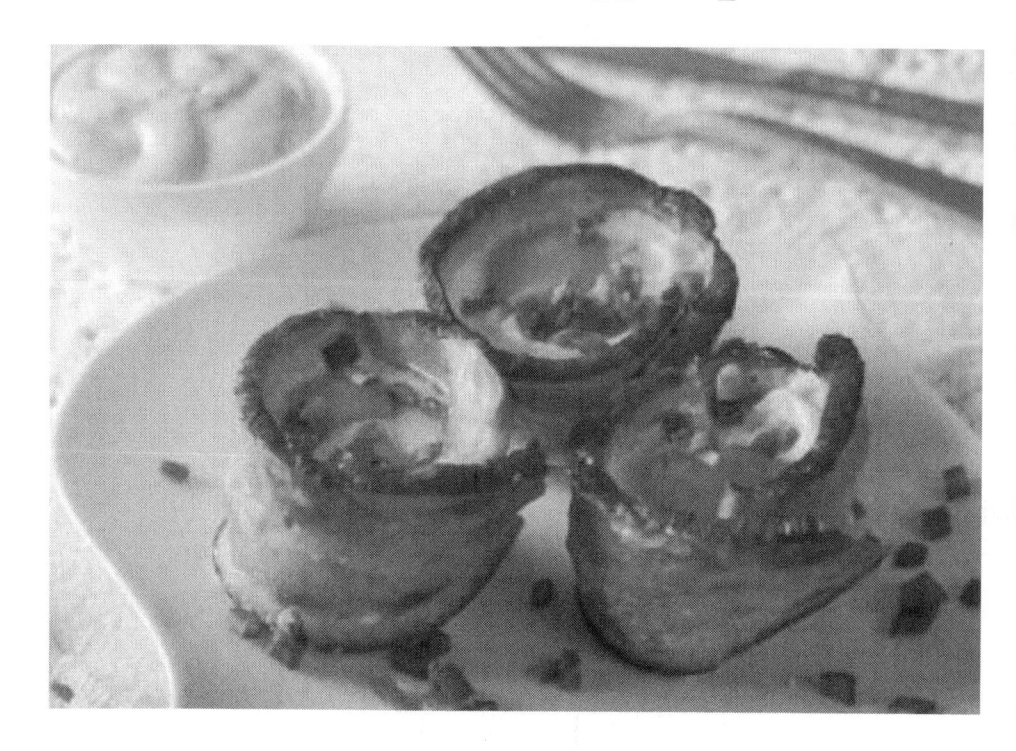

Nutrition Facts Per Serving

Calories	Fats	Proteins	Carbohydrates
128.1	9.7	9.6	0.6

Ingredients

Serves	1	2	3	4	5	6	7	8
Bacon slice	1	2	3	4	5	6	7	8
Egg, at room temperature	1	2	3	4	5	6	7	8
Salt, by taste								
Black pepper, by taste								

Instructions

1. Switch on the oven, then set it to 400 degrees F, and let it preheat.
2. In the meantime, place a frying pan over medium heat and when hot, place a bacon slice and then cook for 2 to 3 minutes per side until tender-crisp.
3. Remove the bacon from the pan, pat dry with a paper towel, cut it in half, and then arrange the slices into a silicone muffin, so that they cover the sides and bottom of the cup.
4. Crack the egg into the prepared muffin cup, sprinkle salt and black pepper on top, and then bake for 7 minutes or more until the egg has cooked to the desired doneness and the bacon is crispy.
5. Serve immediately.

Cheesy Avocado Egg Boat

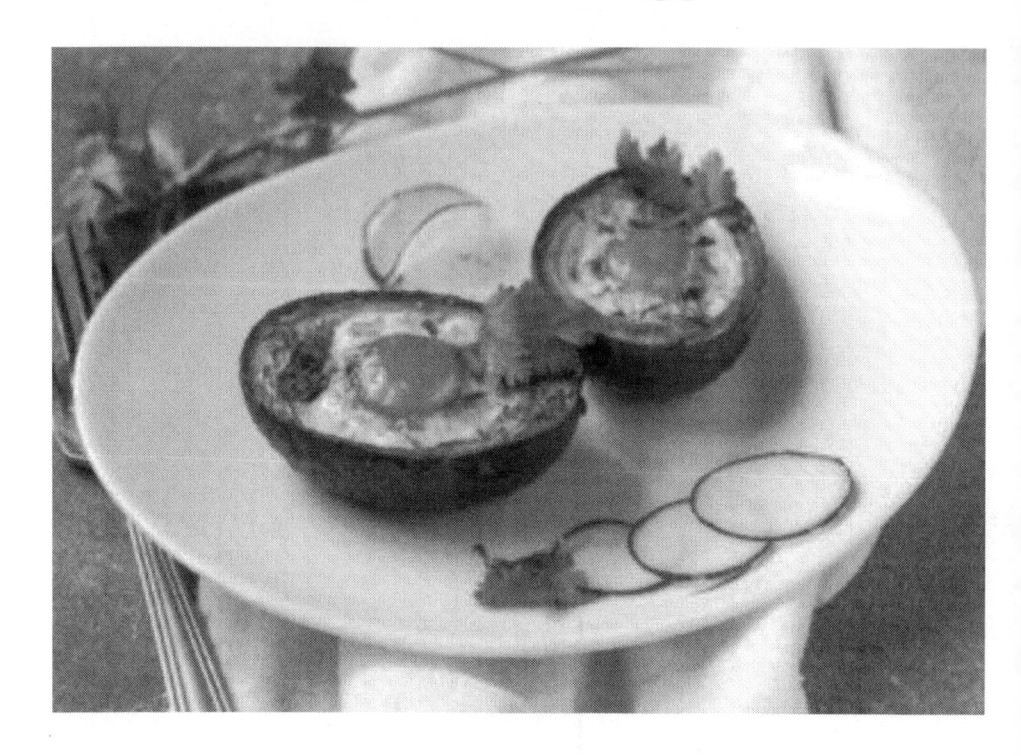

Nutrition Facts Per Serving

Calories	Fats	Proteins	Carbohydrates
528	45.8	22.4	6.6

Ingredients

Serves	1	2	3	4	5	6	7	8
Avocado, pitted	½	1	1 ½	2	2 ½	3	3 ½	4
Egg, at room temperature	1	2	3	4	5	6	7	8
Bacon, cooked, chopped, tablespoon	1	2	3	4	5	6	7	8
Cheddar cheese, grated, full fat	1	2	3	4	5	6	7	8
Salt, by taste								
Black pepper, by taste								

Instructions

1. Switch on the oven, then set it to 400 degrees F, and let it preheat.
2. In the meantime, scoop out some flesh from the avocado half and then crack the egg in it.
3. Sprinkle the bacon on top of the egg, season with salt and black pepper, sprinkle with cheese, and then bake for 10 to 12 minutes until the egg yolks have cooked.
4. Serve directly.

Cauliflower Hash Browns

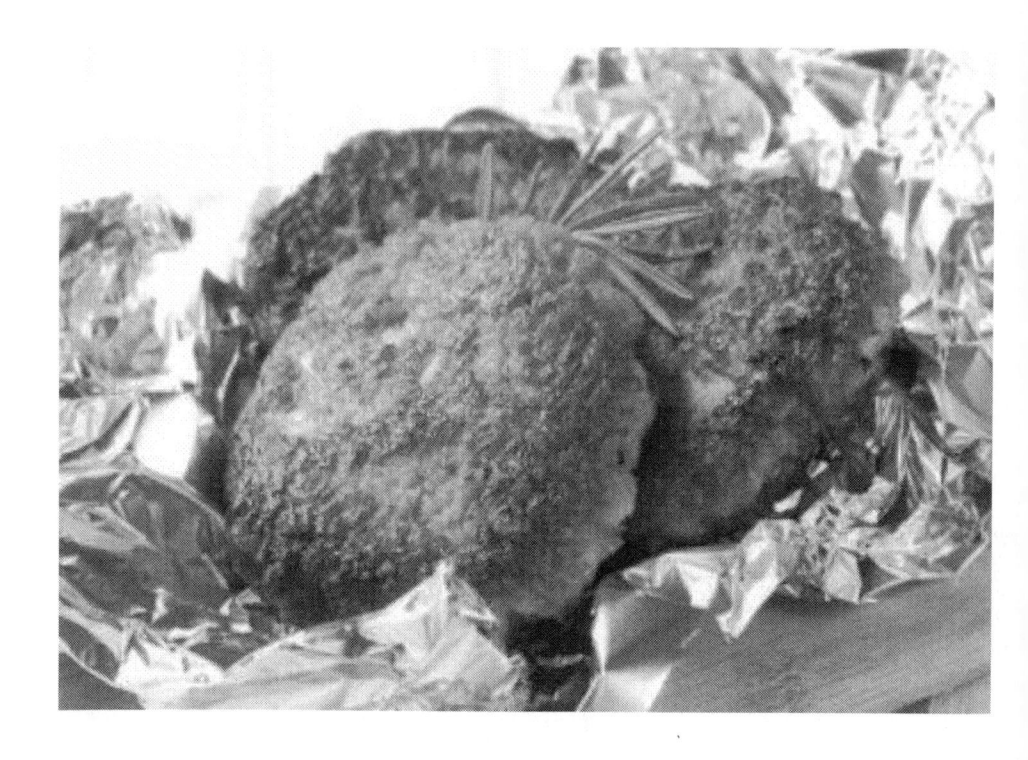

Nutrition Facts Per Serving

Calories	Fats	Proteins	Carbohydrates
282	25.7	9.2	3.5

Ingredients

Serves	1	2	3	4	5	6	7	8
Grated cauliflower, cup	½	1	1 ½	2	2 ½	3	3 ½	4
Bacon slice	2	4	6	8	10	12	14	16
Garlic powder	¼	½	¾	1	1 ¼	1 ½	1 ¾	2
Avocado oil	1	2	3	4	5	6	7	8
Salt, teaspoon	½	1	1 ½	2	2 ½	3	3 ½	4
Black pepper, teaspoon	1/8	¼	1/3	½	2/3	¾	1	1 1/8

Instructions

1. Take a medium microwave-proof bowl, place the grated cauliflower in it, and then cover with some plastic wrap.
2. Poke some holes in the plastic wrap, microwave for 3 to 4 minutes until tender, and when done, uncover the bowl and then drain it well.
3. Wrap the cauliflower in a cheesecloth and then twist it thoroughly to drain any moisture from the cauliflower as much as possible.
4. Crack the egg in a medium bowl, add salt, black pepper, and garlic, whisk until blended, and then stir in cauliflower until combined.
5. Place the oil in a medium skillet pan, place it over medium heat and when hot, scoop cauliflower mixture in it, ¼ cup of mixture per hash brown and then shape it like a hash brown.
6. Cook the hash browns for 4 to 5 minutes per side until golden brown and crisp and then transfer to the plate.
7. Place the bacon slices into the pan, cook it for 2 to 3 minutes per side until crisp and then transfer to the plate containing the hash browns.
8. Serve ASAP.

Bell Pepper Eggs

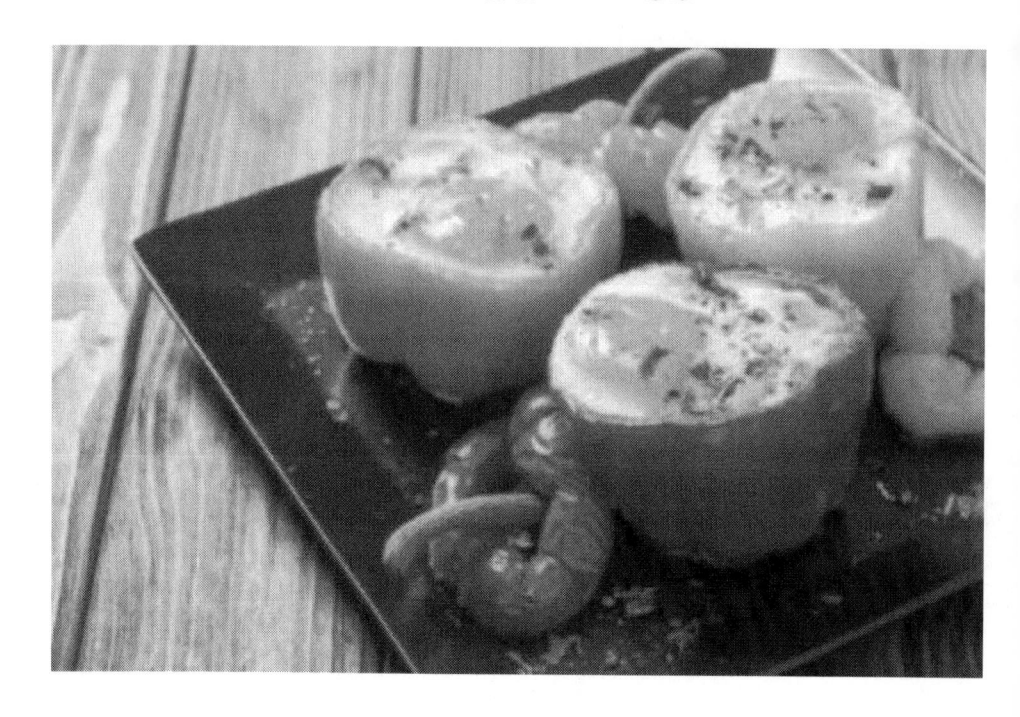

Nutrition Facts Per Serving

Calories	Fats	Proteins	Carbohydrates
124	9.9	7.1	1.6

Ingredients

Serves	1	2	3	4	5	6	7	8
Bell pepper, any color	1	2	3	4	5	6	7	8
Egg, at room temperature	1	2	3	4	5	6	7	8
Salt, by taste								
Black pepper, by taste								

Instructions

1. Switch on the oven, then set it to 400 degrees F, and let it preheat.
2. In the meantime, remove the top from the pepper, remove the seeds and core, spray the pepper inside out with avocado oil spray, and then crack the egg in it.
3. Place the prepared paper in a baking dish and then bake for 10 to 12 minutes until the egg has set. Lastly, cook to the desired level.
4. When done, sprinkle salt and black pepper over the egg and then serve.

Cinnamon Muffin

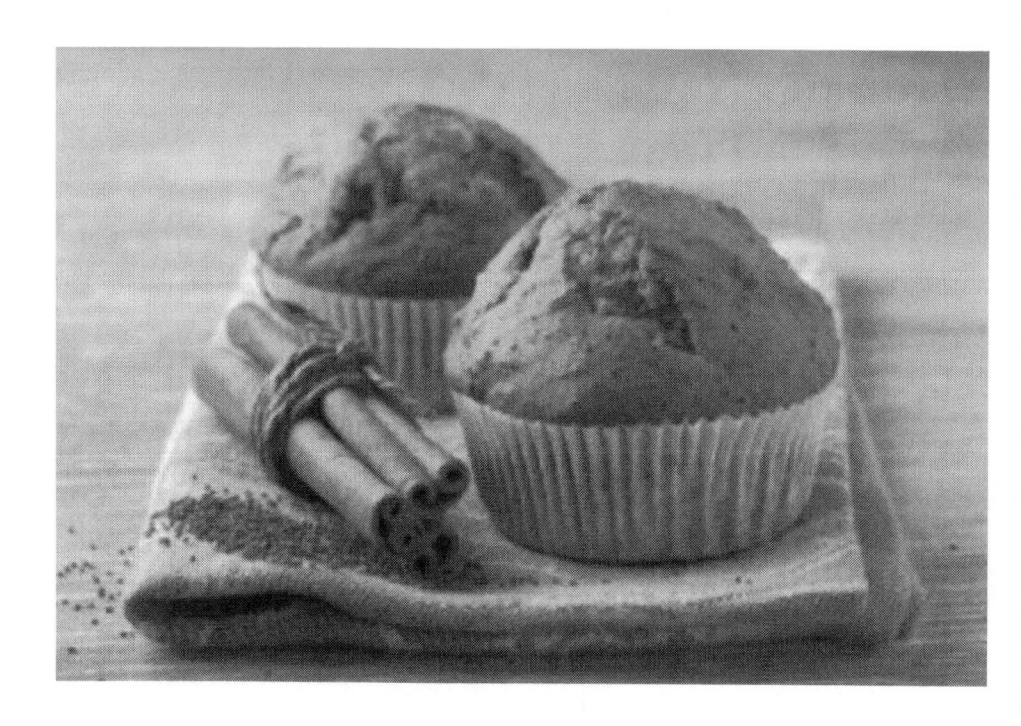

Nutrition Facts Per Serving

Calories	Fats	Proteins	Carbohydrates
269	27.1	4.9	2.6

Ingredients

Serves	1	2	3	4	5	6	7	8
Heavy cream, full-fat, tablespoon	2/3	1 1/3	2	2 2/3	3 1/3	4	4 2/3	5 1/3
Butter, unsalted, tablespoon	½	1	1 ½	2	2 ½	3	3 ½	4
Egg, pasteurized	¼	½	¾	1	1 ¼	1 ½	1 ¾	2
Erythritol sweetener, tablespoon	2/3	1 1/3	2	2 2/3	3 1/3	4	4 2/3	5 1/3
Almond flour, tablespoon	2	4	6	8	10	12	14	16
Ground cinnamon, teaspoon	1/16	1/8	1/4	1/3	½	2/3	¾	1

Instructions

1. Switch on the oven, then set it to 375 degrees F, and let it preheat.
2. Take a medium bowl, place the egg and cream in it, and then whisk until blended.
3. Add the remaining ingredients, stir until smooth, and then pour the mixture into a greased silicone muffin cup.
4. Bake it for 15 minutes until firm and the top turn golden brown, and when done, let the muffin rest for 5 minutes before taking it out to cool completely.
5. Serve swiftly.

Beef and Spinach Frittata

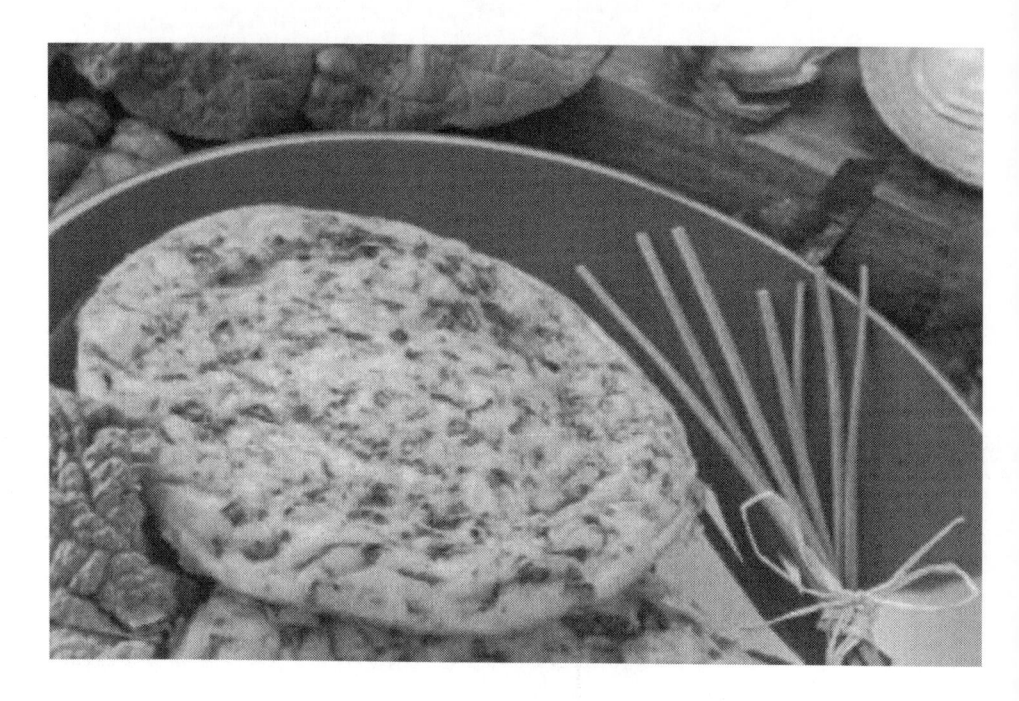

Nutrition Facts Per Serving

Calories	Fats	Proteins	Carbohydrates
504	33.6	45.4	5

Ingredients

Serves	1	2	3	4	5	6	7	8
Ground beef, grass-fed, ounces	4	8	12	16	20	24	28	32
Chopped spinach, fresh, ounces	3	6	9	12	15	18	21	24
Minced garlic, teaspoon	1/4	1/2	3/4	1	1 1/4	1 1/2	1 3/4	2
Avocado oil, teaspoon	1	2	3	4	5	6	7	8
Eggs, at room temperature	2	4	6	8	10	12	14	16
Salt, by taste	1/3	2/3	1	1 1/3	1 2/3	2	2 1/3	2 2/3
Black pepper, by taste	1/4	1/2	3/4	1	1 1/4	1 1/2	1 3/4	2

Instructions

1. Switch on the oven, then set it to 400 degrees F, and let it preheat.
2. In the meantime, place the oil in a medium skillet pan over medium heat and when hot, add the spinach and cook it for 3 to 4 minutes until spinach wilts.
3. Then spoon the spinach to a bowl, wipe clean the pan, return it over medium heat, and keep it hot.
4. Add the beef, cook it for 8 to 10 minutes until cooked, stir in the spinach, salt, and black pepper until combined and cook for 1 minute until hot.
5. Then remove the pan from heat and spread the beef mixture evenly.
6. Crack the eggs in a small bowl, add salt and black pepper, whisk until blended and then pour the eggs over the spinach mixture.
7. Bake the frittata in the oven for 10 to 12 minutes until cooked and the top turns golden brown.
8. When done, let the frittata cool for 5 minutes, cut it into slices, and then serve.

Eggs in Clouds

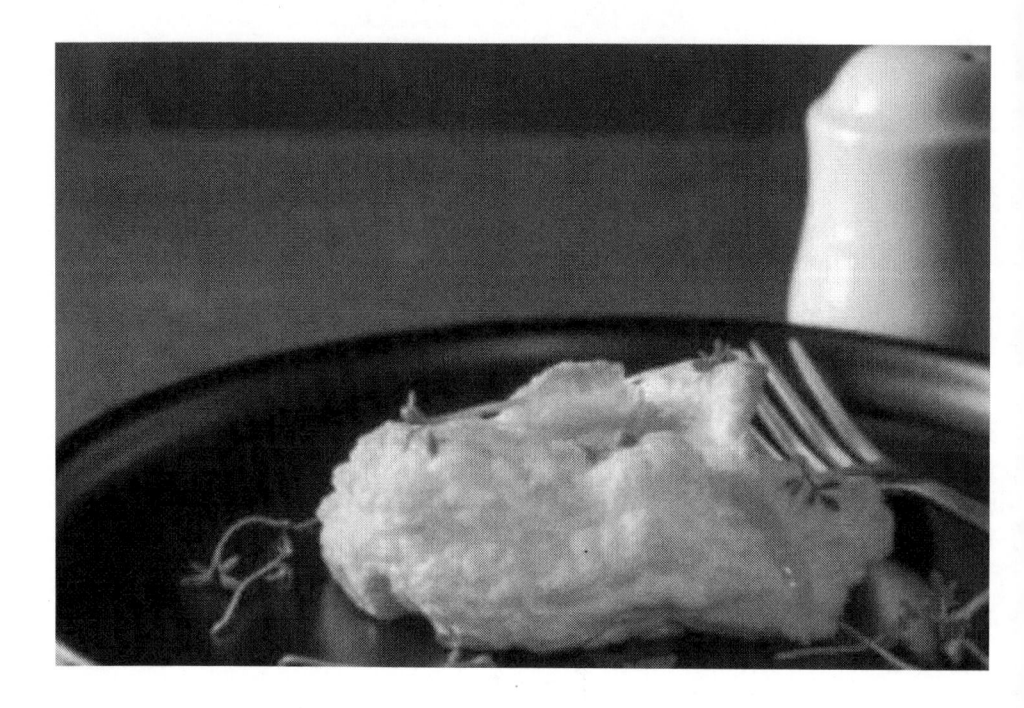

Nutrition Facts Per Serving

Calories	Fats	Proteins	Carbohydrates
183	15.5	10.1	0.9

Ingredients

Serves	1	2	3	4	5	6	7	8
Eggs, at room temperature	1	2	3	4	5	6	7	8
Bacon slice	1	2	3	4	5	6	7	8
Salt, by taste								
Black pepper, by taste								

Instructions

1. Switch on the oven, then set it to 350 degrees F, and let it preheat.
2. In the meantime, place a frying pan over medium heat and when hot, place the bacon slice on it and then cook for 3 minutes per side until crisp.
3. Transfer the bacon to a cutting board, cool it for 5 minutes, and then chop it.
4. Separate the egg yolk and egg white between two bowls, beat the egg white until stiff peaks form, and then fold in the chopped bacon.
5. Take a small baking sheet, line it with parchment sheet or foil, spoon the bacon mixture on it like a mound, and then make a well in it.
6. Bake it for 3 minutes, then place the egg yolk in the well, and bake for another 2 minutes.
7. When done, sprinkle salt and black pepper over the egg and then serve.

Bagel

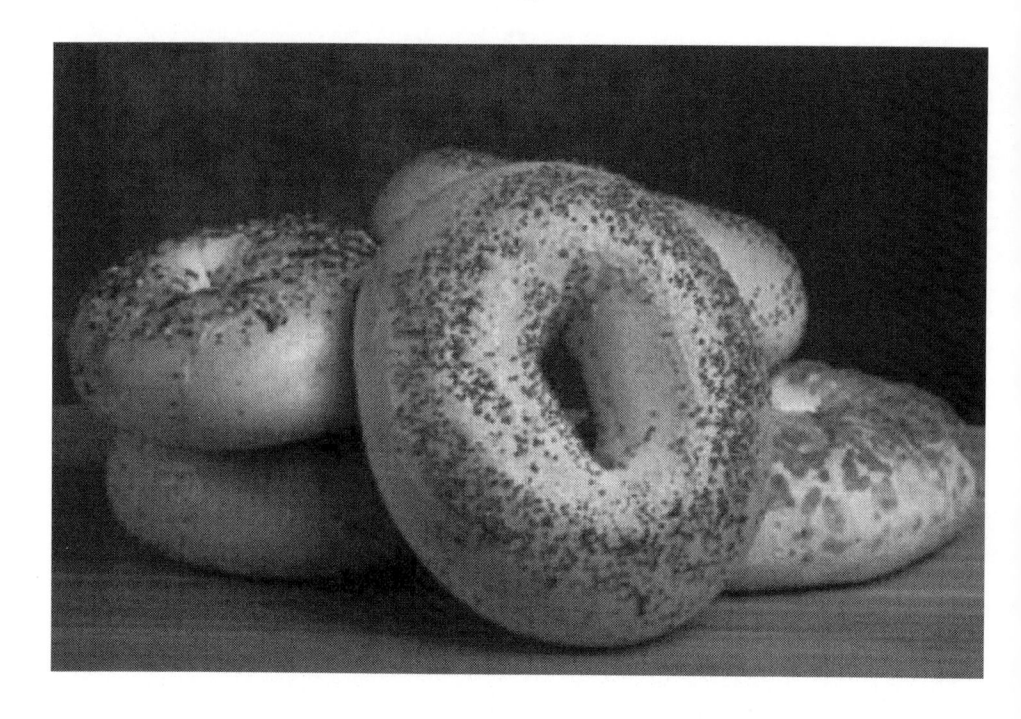

Nutrition Facts Per Serving

Calories	Fats	Proteins	Carbohydrates
268	20.1	19.9	1.4

Ingredients

Serves	1	2	3	4	5	6	7	8
Ground beef, grass-fed, ounces	2	4	6	8	10	12	14	16
Bacon slice	1	2	3	4	5	6	7	8
Egg, at room temperature	1	2	3	4	5	6	7	8
Tomato sauce, tablespoon	1	2	3	4	5	6	7	8
Paprika, teaspoon	¼	½	¾	1	1 ¼	1 ½	1 ¾	2
Salt, teaspoon	¼	½	¾	1	1 ¼	1 ½	1 ¾	2
Black pepper, teaspoon	¼	½	¾	1	1 ¼	1 ½	1 ¾	2

Instructions

1. Switch on the oven, set it to 400 degrees F, and let it preheat.
2. In the meantime, chop the bacon and add to a medium bowl.
3. Add the remaining ingredients, stir until well combined, and then shape the mixture into a bagel.
4. Arrange the bagel on a baking dish, and then bake it for 15 to 20 minutes until thoroughly cooked, turning halfway.
5. When done, let the bagel cool for 5 minutes, then slice it in half lengthwise and serve.

Cream Cheese Pancake

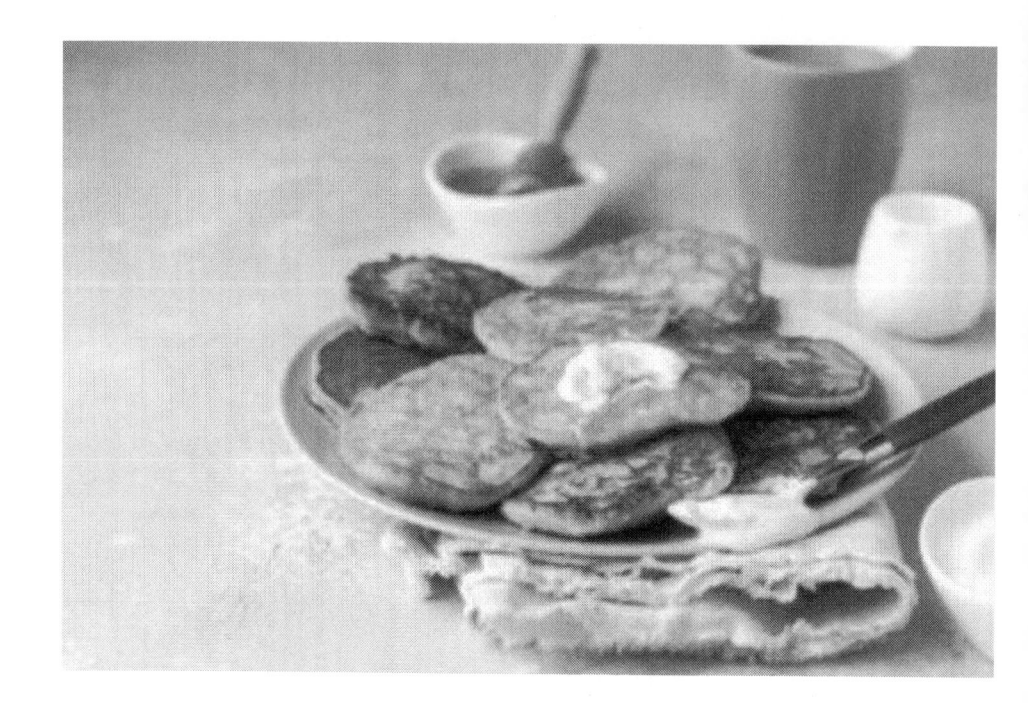

Nutrition Facts Per Serving

Calories	Fats	Proteins	Carbohydrates
245.3	16.9	20.8	2.5

Ingredients

Serves	1	2	3	4	5	6	7	8
Cream cheese, full-fat, ounces	2	4	6	8	10	12	14	16
Eggs, at room temperature	2	4	6	8	10	12	14	16
Cinnamon, ground, teaspoon	½	1	1 ½	2	2 ½	3	3 ½	4
Butter, unsalted, teaspoon	1	2	3	4	5	6	7	8

Instructions

1. Crack eggs in a blender, add cinnamon and cream cheese, blend for 30 seconds until smooth, and then let the mixture rest for 5 minutes.
2. Place the butter in a medium skillet pan over medium heat, and let it melt.
3. Ladle the cream cheese mixture into the pan, one-fourth mixture per pancake, shape the mixture into a pancake, and then cook for 2 to 3 minutes per side until golden brown.
4. Serve promptly.

Mozzarella and Garlic Waffles

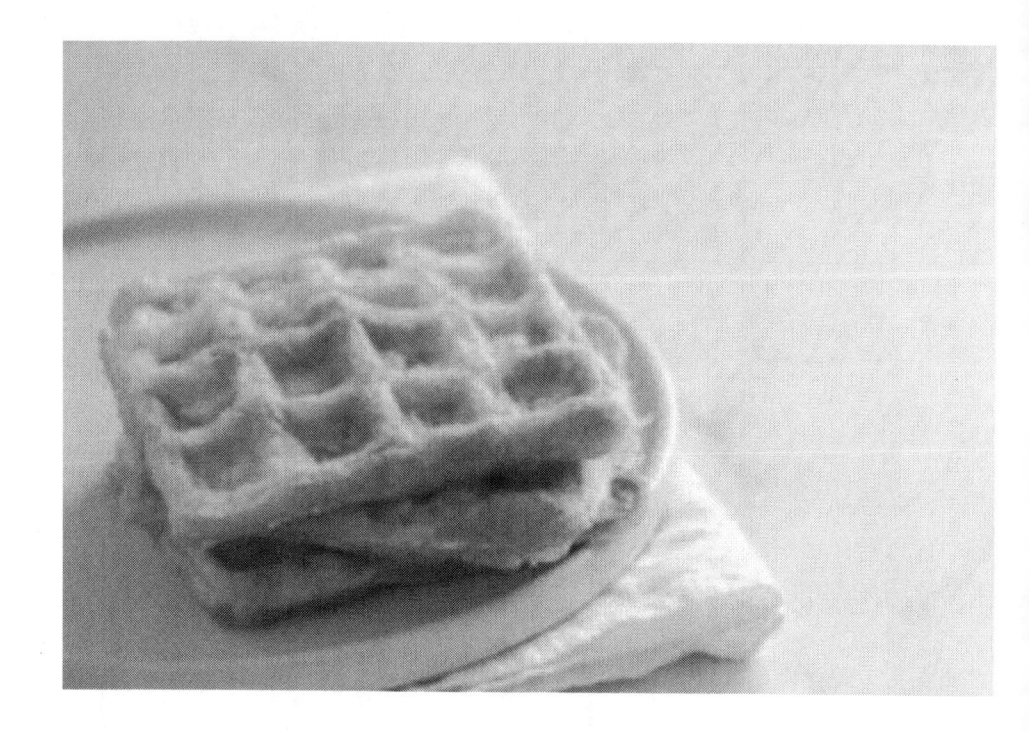

Nutrition Facts Per Serving

Calories	Fats	Proteins	Carbohydrates
260.4	18.8	20.2	2.6

Ingredients

Serves	1	2	3	4	5	6	7	8
Baking powder, teaspoon	¼	½	¾	1	1 ¼	1 ½	1 ¾	2
Minced garlic, teaspoon	½	1	1 ½	2	2 ½	3	3 ½	4
Egg, at room temperature	1	2	3	4	5	6	7	8
Mozzarella cheese, grated, full-fat, cup	½	1	1 ½	2	2 ½	3	3 ½	4
Italian seasoning, teaspoon	½	1	1 ½	2	2 ½	3	3 ½	4

Instructions

1. Turn on a waffle maker and then set it for preheating.
2. In the meantime, place all the ingredients in a medium bowl and then whisk well by using an immersion blender until smooth batter comes together.
3. Ladle the waffle batter into the hot waffle maker and then cook it for 3 to 5 minutes until firm and the waffle turns golden brown.
4. Serve directly.

Porridge

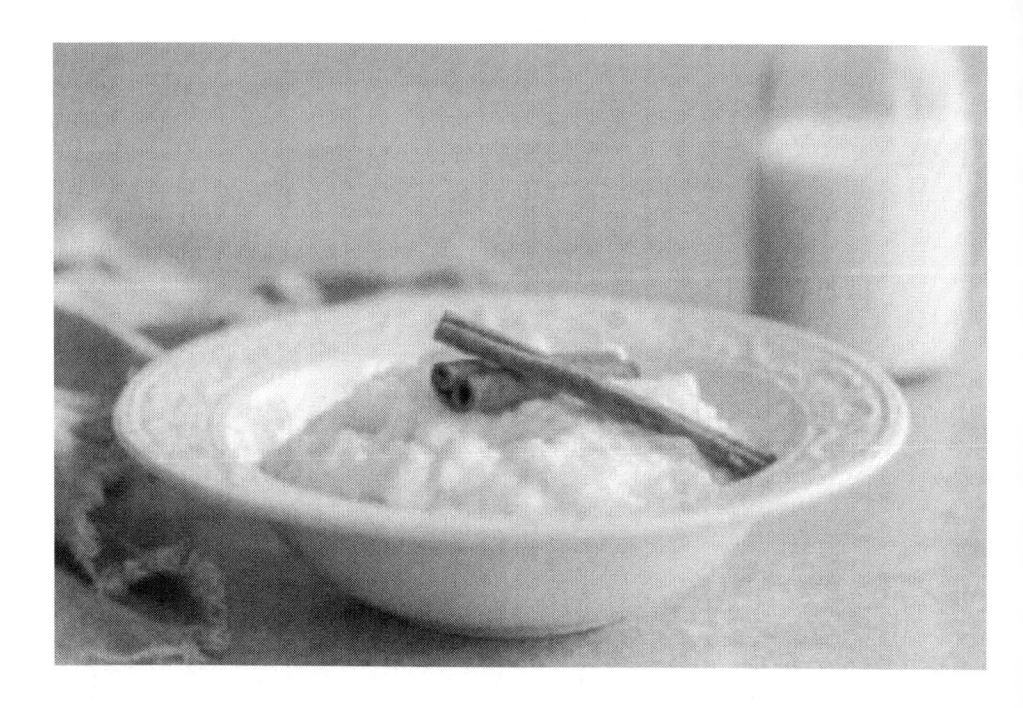

Nutrition Facts Per Serving

Calories	Fats	Proteins	Carbohydrates
681	64.3	17	8.5

Ingredients

Serves	1	2	3	4	5	6	7	8
Coconut flour, tablespoon	1	2	3	4	5	6	7	8
Psyllium husk powder, teaspoon	¼	½	¾	1	1 ¼	1 ½	1 ¾	2
Egg, at room temperature	1	2	3	4	5	6	7	8
Heavy cream, full-fat, ounces	3	6	9	12	15	18	21	24
Butter, unsalted, ounces	1	2	3	4	5	6	7	8

Instructions

1. Crack the eggs in a medium bowl, add the husk powder and flour in it, and then whisk until smooth.
2. Place a small microwave-oven proof bowl, place cream and butter in it, and then microwave for 45 seconds or more until butter melts, stirring every 20 seconds.
3. Stir the butter mixture into the flour mixture until creamy and then top with favorite keto fruits or nuts.
4. Serve punctually.

Jalapeno Waffle

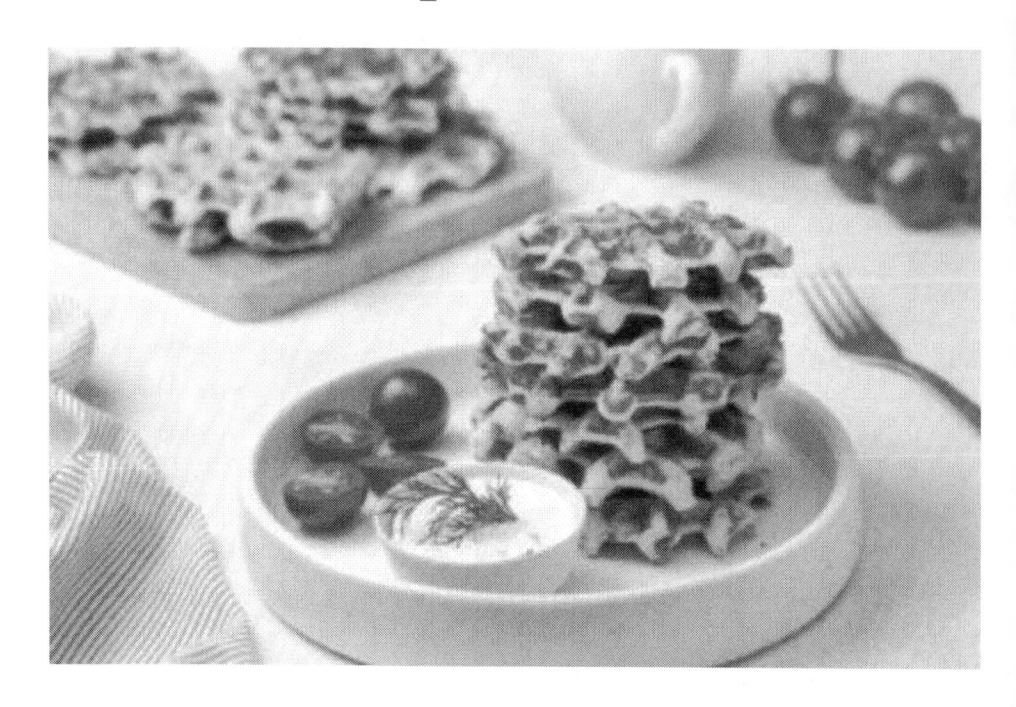

Nutrition Facts Per Serving

Calories	Fats	Proteins	Carbohydrates
294.7	23.9	15.9	4

Ingredients

Serves	1	2	3	4	5	6	7	8
Coconut flour, teaspoon	2	4	6	8	10	12	14	16
Chopped jalapeno, tablespoon	½	1	1 ½	2	2 ½	3	3 ½	4
Cream cheese, softened, tablespoon	2	4	6	8	10	12	14	16
Egg, at room temperature	1	2	3	4	5	6	7	8
Mozzarella cheese, grated, full-fat, ounces	2	4	6	8	10	12	14	16
Salt, teaspoon	¼	½	¾	1	1 ¼	1 ½	1 ¾	2

Instructions

1. Turn on a waffle maker and then set it for preheating.
2. In the meantime, place all the ingredients in a medium bowl, and then whisk well by using an immersion blender until a smooth batter form.
3. Ladle the waffle batter into the hot waffle maker and then cook it for 3 to 5 minutes until firm and waffle turn golden brown.
4. Serve swiftly.

Breakfast Vanilla Pudding

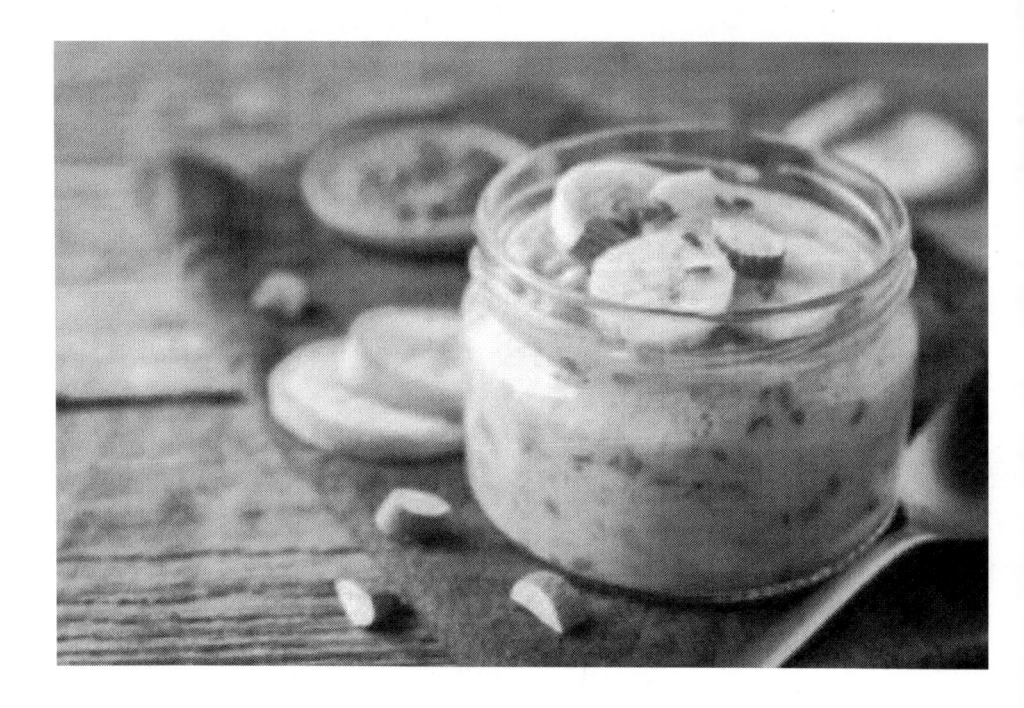

Nutrition Facts Per Serving

Calories	Fats	Proteins	Carbohydrates
288	27	4	8

Ingredients

Serves	1	2	3	4	5	6	7	8
Heavy cream, full-fat, tablespoon	2	4	6	8	10	12	14	16
Coconut milk, unsweetened, full-fat, cup	¼	½	¾	1	1 ¼	1 ½	1 ¾	2
Chia seeds, tablespoon	1 ¼	2 ½	3 ¾	5	6 ¼	7 ½	8 ¾	10
Vanilla extract, unsweetened, teaspoon	½	1	1 ½	2	2 ½	3	3 ½	4
Erythritol sweetener, teaspoon	1	2	3	4	5	6	7	8

Instructions

1. Take a medium bowl, place all the ingredients, and then stir until combined.
2. Cover the bowl with its lid and then let the pudding rest in the refrigerator for 30 minutes until thickened.
3. Stir the pudding and then serve.

Waffles with Poached Eggs

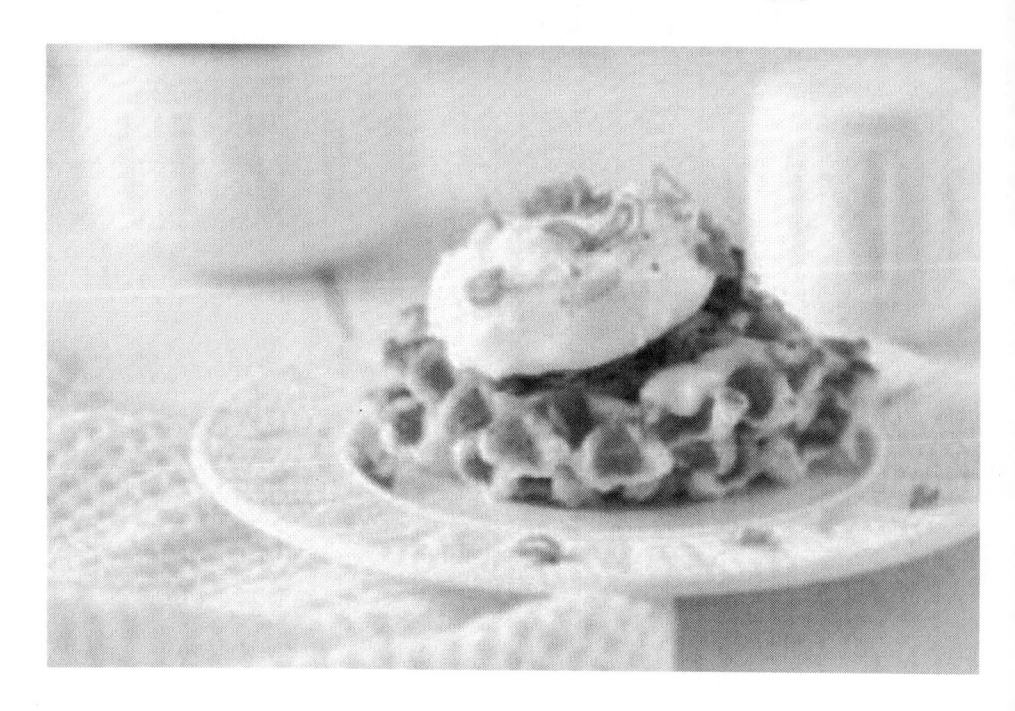

Nutrition Facts Per Serving

Calories	Fats	Proteins	Carbohydrates
279	20.5	20.2	3.5

Ingredients

Serves	1	2	3	4	5	6	7	8
Coconut flour, teaspoon	1	2	3	4	5	6	7	8
Cheddar cheese, grated, full-fat, cup	1/4	1/2	3/4	1	1 1/4	1 1/2	1 3/4	2
Egg, at room temperature	2	4	6	8	10	12	14	16
Salt, teaspoon	1/8	1/4	1/3	1/2	2/3	3/4	1	1 1/8
Black pepper, teaspoon	1/8	1/4	1/3	1/2	2/3	3/4	1	1 1/8

Instructions

1. Turn on a waffle maker and then set it for preheating.
2. In the meantime, place flour in a medium bowl, add cheese and 1 egg, and then whisk well by using an immersion blender until a smooth batter comes together.
3. Ladle the waffle batter into the hot waffle maker and then cook it for 3 to 5 minutes until firm and the waffle becomes golden brown.
4. When done, transfer the waffle to a plate and set aside until required.
5. Take a small pot, fill it half full with water, and then bring it to boil over medium heat.
6. Crack the egg in a large spoon or ramekin, carefully transfer the egg into the water, and then cook it for 3 to 4 minutes until done.
7. Use a slotted spoon to remove the poached egg from the pot and then place it on top of the waffle.
8. Sprinkle salt and black pepper over a poached egg and then serve.

Pumpkin Spiced Hemp Porridge

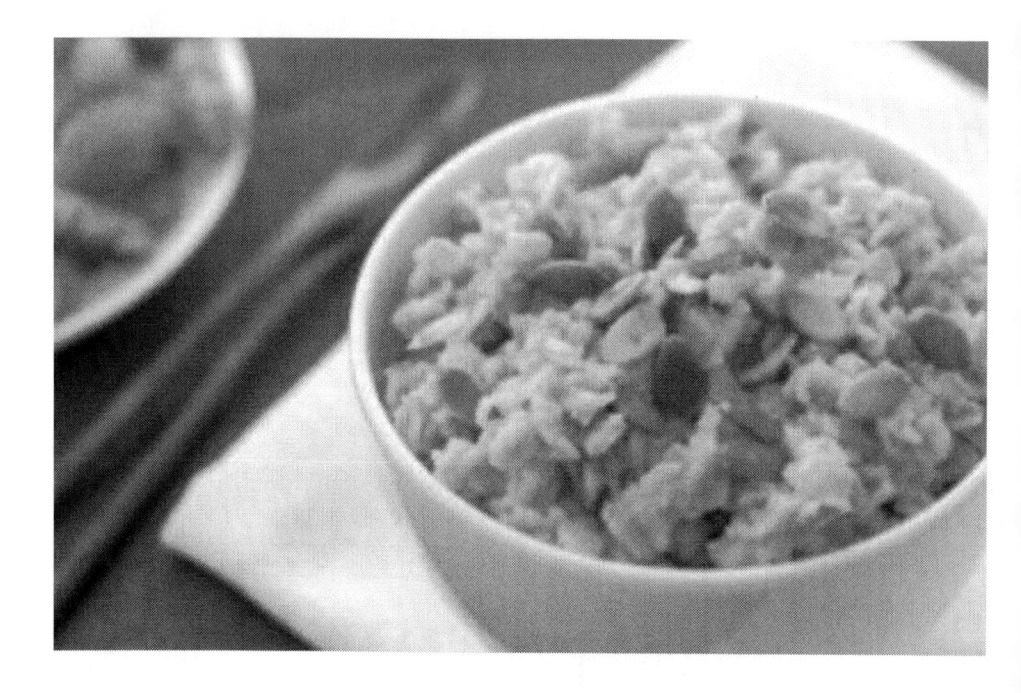

Nutrition Facts Per Serving

Calories	Fats	Proteins	Carbohydrates
575	48.6	27.2	5.4

Ingredients

Serves	1	2	3	4	5	6	7	8
Hemp hearts, cup	½	1	2 ½	3	3 ½	4	4 ½	5
Water, cup	½	1	1 ½	2	2 ½	3	3 ½	4
Almond milk, full-fat, unsweetened, cup	¾	1 ½	2 ¼	3	3 ¾	4 ½	5 ¼	6
Coconut cream, full-fat, tablespoon	2	4	6	8	10	12	14	16
Pumpkin spice, teaspoon	1/8	¼	1/3	½	2/3	¾	1	1 1/8
Ground cinnamon, teaspoon	½	1	1 ½	2	2 ½	3	3 ½	4
Erythritol sweetener, tablespoon	1	2	3	4	5	6	7	8

Instructions

1. Pour milk in a small pan, place it over medium-high heat, and add water, sweetener, cinnamon, and pumpkin spice.
2. Stir until smooth, and then bring the mixture to a boil.
3. Stir in hemp hearts until mixed, switch heat to medium-low level, and cook it for 35 minutes until a thick and creamy mixture emerges.
4. When done, remove the pan from heat, taste to adjust the spice and sweetener, and then stir in cream until combined.
5. Serve directly.

Breakfast Tuna Wrap

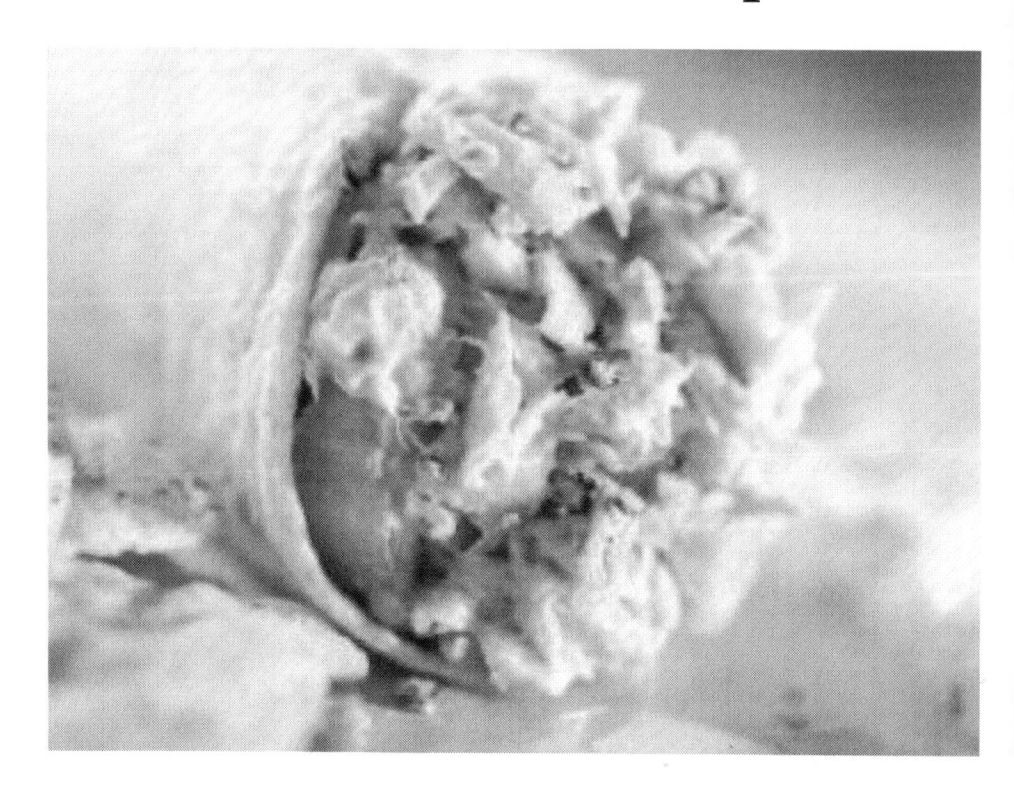

Nutrition Facts Per Serving

Calories	Fats	Proteins	Carbohydrates
321.5	28.6	15.3	1

Ingredients

Serves	1	2	3	4	5	6	7	8
Tuna, canned, drained, ounces	2	4	6	8	10	12	14	16
Cayenne pepper, teaspoon	1/8	1/4	1/3	½	2/3	3/4	1	1 1/8
Mayonnaise, tablespoon	2	4	6	8	10	12	14	16
Avocado oil, teaspoon	1	2	3	4	5	6	7	8
Egg, at room temperature	1	2	3	4	5	6	7	8
Salt, teaspoon	1/8	1/4	1/3	½	2/3	3/4	1	1 1/8
Black pepper, teaspoon	1/8	1/4	1/3	½	2/3	3/4	1	1 1/8

Instructions

1. Crack the egg in a small bowl, add salt and black pepper, and then whisk until frothy.
2. Place the oil in a frying pan over medium heat, and when hot, pour the egg in it, spread it evenly by rotating the pan, and then cook it for 2 minutes per side until done.
3. When done, transfer the egg to a plate.
4. Place the tuna in a small bowl, add cayenne pepper, stir in mayonnaise until well mixed, and then spoon it on one side of the egg.
5. Roll the egg to cover the tuna like a wrap and then serve.

Beef Omelet Wrap

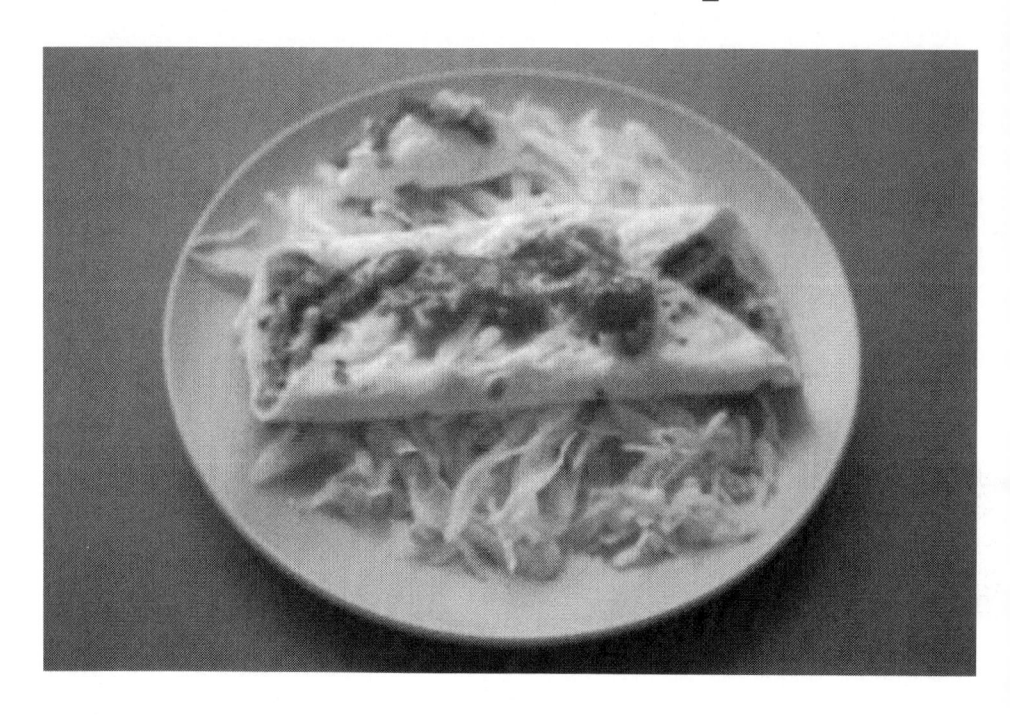

Nutrition Facts Per Serving

Calories	Fats	Proteins	Carbohydrates
295	21.6	24.3	0.7

Ingredients

Serves	1	2	3	4	5	6	7	8
Ground beef, grass-fed, ounces	2	4	6	8	10	12	14	16
Egg, at room temperature	1	2	3	4	5	6	7	8
Heavy cream, full-fat, tablespoon	1	2	3	4	5	6	7	8
Mozzarella cheese, grated, full-fat, tablespoon	1	2	3	4	5	6	7	8
Salt, teaspoon	1/8	1/4	1/3	½	2/3	3/4	1	1 1/8
Black pepper, teaspoon	1/8	1/4	1/3	½	2/3	3/4	1	1 1/8

Instructions

1. Place a medium skillet pan over medium heat and when hot, add the beef and then cook for 7 to 10 minutes until thoroughly cooked.
2. When done, transfer the beef to a bowl and set aside until required.
3. Crack the egg in a small bowl, add cream, salt, and black pepper and then whisk until blended.
4. Pour the egg into the pan, spread it evenly by rotating the pan, and then cook for 2 minutes per side until firm.
5. Transfer the egg to a plate, spread beef on its one side, and then roll the egg to cover the beef like a wrap.
6. Serve promptly.

Peanut Butter Oatmeal

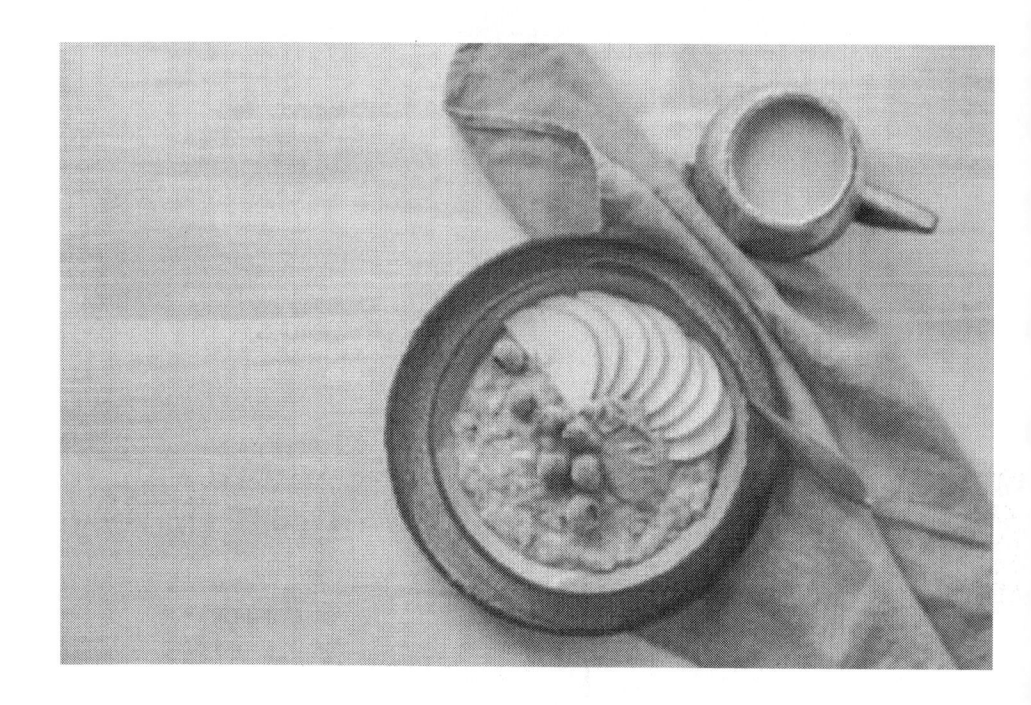

Nutrition Facts Per Serving

Calories	Fats	Proteins	Carbohydrates
250	22	10	3

Ingredients

Serves	1	2	3	4	5	6	7	8
Coconut flakes, unsweetened, cup	½	1	1 ½	2	2 ½	3	3 ½	4
Hemp seeds, cup	¼	½	¾	1	1 ¼	1 ½	1 ¾	2
Coconut flour, tablespoon	1	2	3	4	5	6	7	8
Coconut milk, full-fat, unsweetened, cup	½	1	1 ½	2	2 ½	3	3 ½	4
Peanut butter, unsalted, tablespoon	1	2	3	4	5	6	7	8
Water, cup	½	1	1 ½	2	2 ½	3	3 ½	4

Instructions

1. Place the flour in a small saucepan, add hemp seeds and coconut, pour in milk and water, and then stir until well combined and smooth.
2. Place the pan over medium heat, bring the oatmeal to boil, and then switch heat to medium-low level, and then cook it for 2 minutes or more until thickened.
3. Then add the peanut butter into the porridge, stir until mixed, and then remove the pan from heat.
4. Spoon the porridge into a bowl, let it cool for 10 minutes, and then serve.

Cheesy Vegetable Frittata

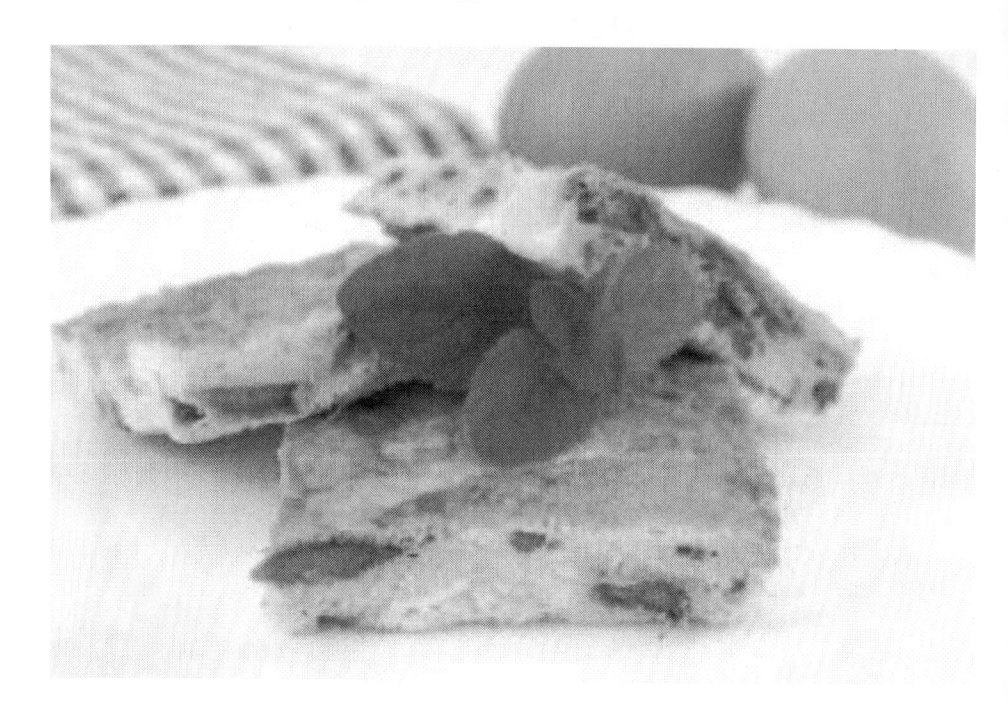

Nutrition Facts Per Serving

Calories	Fats	Proteins	Carbohydrates
347.4	30.5	15.6	2.6

Ingredients

Serves	1	2	3	4	5	6	7	8
Asparagus cuts, ounces	2	4	6	8	10	12	14	16
Garlic powder, teaspoon	1/2	1	1 1/2	2	2 1/2	3	3 1/2	4
Heavy cream, tablespoon	2	4	6	8	10	12	14	16
Egg, at room temperature	2	4	6	8	10	12	14	16
Avocado oil, teaspoons	2	4	6	8	10	12	14	16
Salt, teaspoon	1/4	1/2	3/4	1	1 1/4	1 1/2	1 3/4	2
Black pepper, teaspoon	1/8	1/4	1/3	1/2	2/3	3/4	1	1 1/8

Instructions

1. Switch on the oven, then set it to 350 degrees F, and let it preheat.
2. In the meantime, crack the eggs in a medium bowl, and then add cream, salt, and black pepper.
3. Whisk until combined, add cheese, and then stir until evenly mixed.
4. Place the oil in a medium skillet pan over medium heat; and when hot, add the asparagus and stir until coated in the oil.
5. Sprinkle the garlic powder over asparagus, cook for 4 minutes until asparagus are almost tender and then remove the pan from heat.
6. Spread the asparagus pieces evenly in the pan, pour the egg over them, return the pan over medium-low heat and cook for 2 to 3 minutes until the eggs begin to set.
7. Bake the eggs for 10 minutes or more until firm and the tops turn golden. Finally, when done, let the frittata cool for 5 minutes before cutting it into slices.
8. Serve immediately.

Chicken and Bacon Pancake

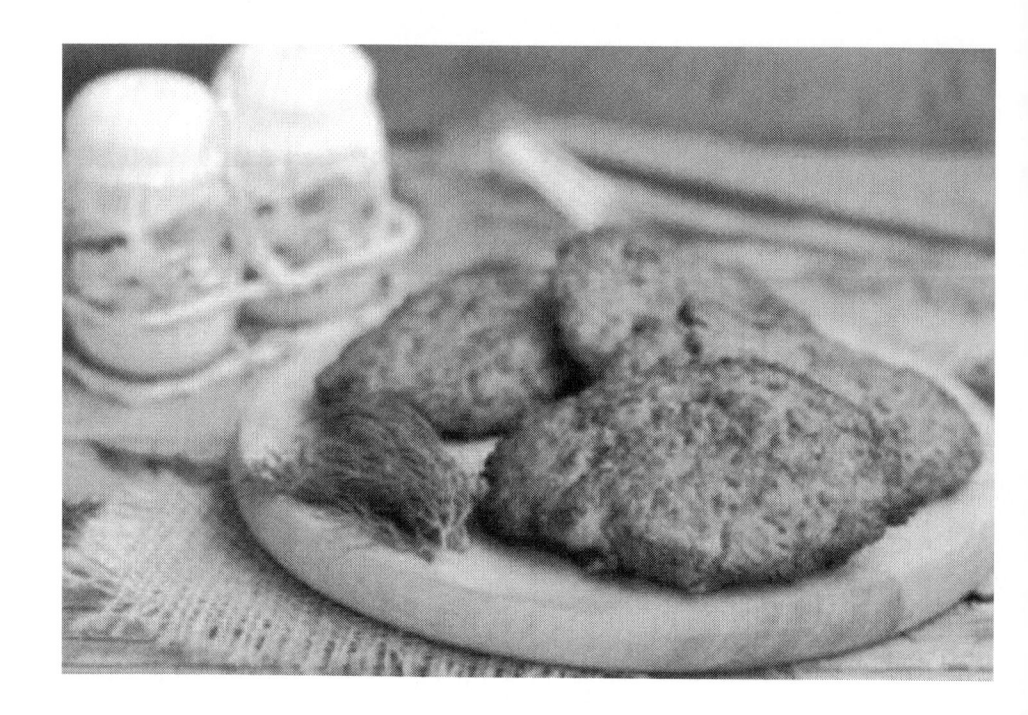

Nutrition Facts Per Serving

Calories	Fats	Proteins	Carbohydrates
594	42.9	49	3

Ingredients

Serves	1	2	3	4	5	6	7	8
Ground chicken, pasteurized, pound	1/3	2/3	1	1 1/3	1 2/3	2	2 1/3	2 2/3
Bacon slice	2	4	6	8	10	12	14	16
Egg, at room temperature	1	2	3	4	5	6	7	8
Avocado oil, tablespoon	1	2	3	4	5	6	7	8
Salt, teaspoon	¼	½	¾	1	1¼	1½	1¾	2
Black pepper, teaspoon	1/8	1/4	1/3	½	2/3	¾	1	1 1/8

Instructions

1. Place the minced chicken in a food processor, add the bacon, salt, black pepper, and egg, and then pulse until well combined.
2. Place the oil in a frying pan over medium heat, and when hot, scoop the chicken mixture in it. Aim for roughly ¼ of the chicken mixture per pancake.
3. Shape the mixture like a pancake and then cook for 5 to 7 minutes per side until nicely browned and cooked.
4. Serve immediately.

Cheesy Garlic Bacon Knots

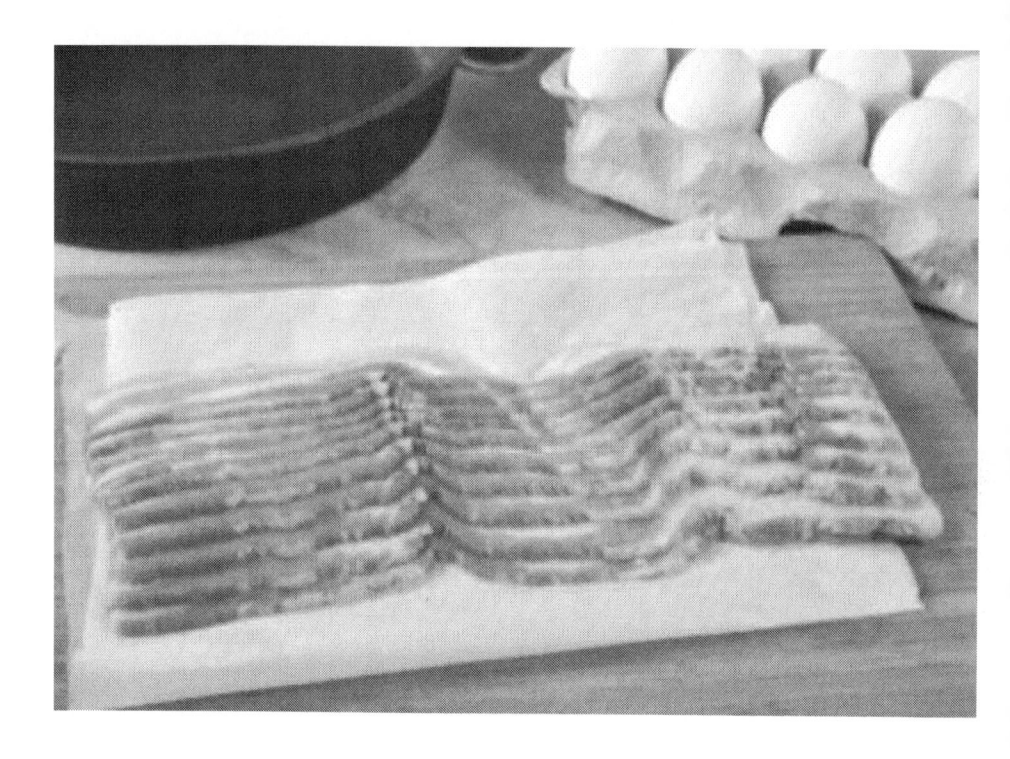

Nutrition Facts Per Serving

Calories	Fats	Proteins	Carbohydrates
308	26.7	15.4	1.5

Ingredients

Serves	1	2	3	4	5	6	7	8
Slices of bacon	4	8	12	16	20	24	28	32
Garlic powder, teaspoon	¼	½	¾	1	1¼	1½	1¾	2
Red pepper flakes, teaspoon	¼	½	¾	1	1¼	1½	1¾	2
Italian seasoning, teaspoon	¼	½	¾	1	1¼	1½	1¾	2
Parmesan cheese, grated, full-fat, tablespoons	2	4	6	8	10	12	14	16

Instructions

1. Switch on the oven, then set it to 425 degrees F, and let it preheat.
2. In the meantime, take a bacon slice, tie it like a double knot, place it on a medium baking sheet, and then repeat with remaining bacon slices.
3. Sprinkle garlic powder, red pepper, and Italian seasoning, and then bake the bacon for 8 to 10 minutes until almost crisp.
4. Remove the baking tray from the oven, sprinkle cheese over them, and then bake for 2 to 3 minutes until the cheese melts.
5. Serve right away.

LUNCH

Cheese Muffin

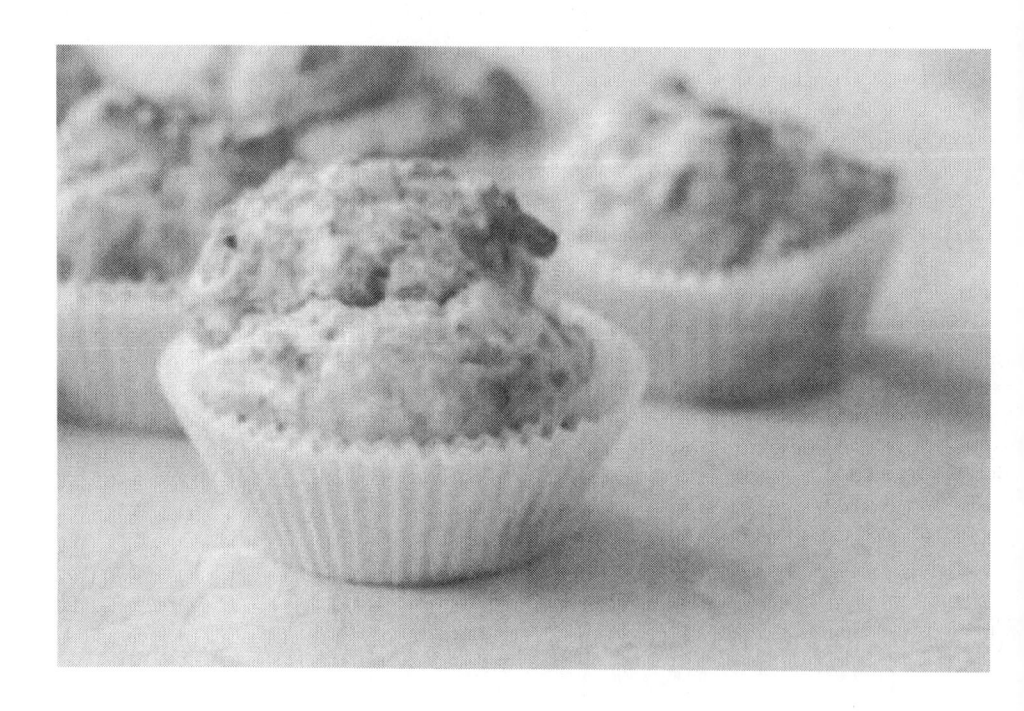

Nutrition Facts Per Serving

Calories	Fats	Proteins	Carbohydrates
240	17.3	18	3

Ingredients

Serves	1	2	3	4	5	6	7	8
Almond flour, teaspoon	4	8	12	16	20	24	28	32
Baking soda, teaspoon	1/16	1/8	¼	1/3	½	2/3	¾	1
Mozzarella cheese, grated, tablespoon	1	2	3	4	5	6	7	8
Parmesan cheese, grated, tablespoon	1	2	3	4	5	6	7	8
Eggs, pasteurized	2	4	6	8	10	12	14	16
Dried basil, teaspoon	½	1	1 ½	2	2 ½	3	3 ½	4
Salt, teaspoon	¼	½	¾	1	1 ¼	1 ½	1 ¾	2

Instructions

1. Crack the eggs in a medium bowl, add the remaining ingredients, and then whisk until combined.
2. Take a large microwave-oven proof silicone muffin, grease it with avocado oil spray, and then spoon the prepared mixture in it.
3. Microwave at a high heat setting for 2 minutes until firm and the top becomes golden. Lastly, serve.

Meat Muffin

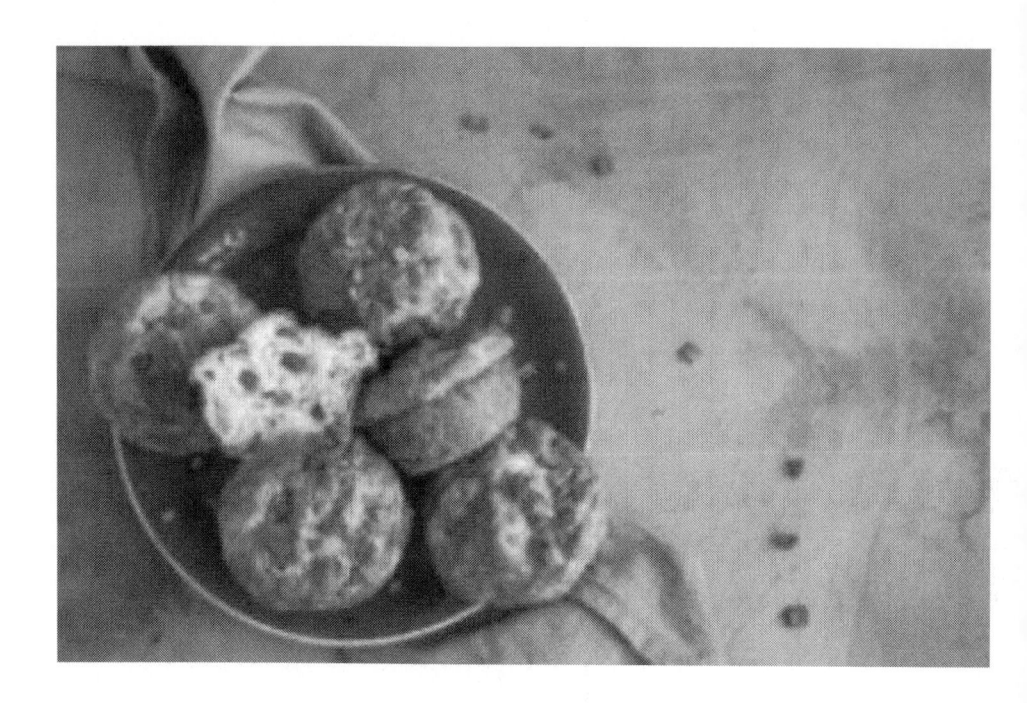

Nutrition Facts Per Serving

Calories	Fats	Proteins	Carbohydrates
194	13	15	1

Ingredients

Serves	1	2	3	4	5	6	7	8
Ground chicken, pasteurized, cup	1/3	2/3	1	1 1/3	1 2/3	2	2 1/3	2 2/3
Cheddar cheese, grated, full-fat, tablespoon	2/3	1 1/3	2	2 2/3	3 1/3	4	4 2/3	5 1/3
Egg, pasteurized	¼	½	¾	1	1 ¼	1 ½	1 ¾	2
Chopped parsley, tablespoon	¼	½	¾	1	1 ¼	1 ½	1 ¾	2
Garlic powder, teaspoon	1/8	¼	1/3	½	2/3	¾	1	1 1/8
Salt, teaspoon	1/8	¼	1/3	½	2/3	¾	1	1 1/8
Black pepper, teaspoon	1/8	¼	1/3	½	2/3	¾	1	1 1/8

Instructions

1. Switch on the oven, then set it to 375 degrees F, and let it preheat.
2. Take a medium bowl, place all the ingredients in it, and then stir until well combined.
3. Take a large silicone muffin cup, spoon mixture in it, and then bake for 10 minutes or more until firm and cooked.
4. When done, remove the muffin from the cup, let it cool slightly, and then serve.

Tuna Egg Boats

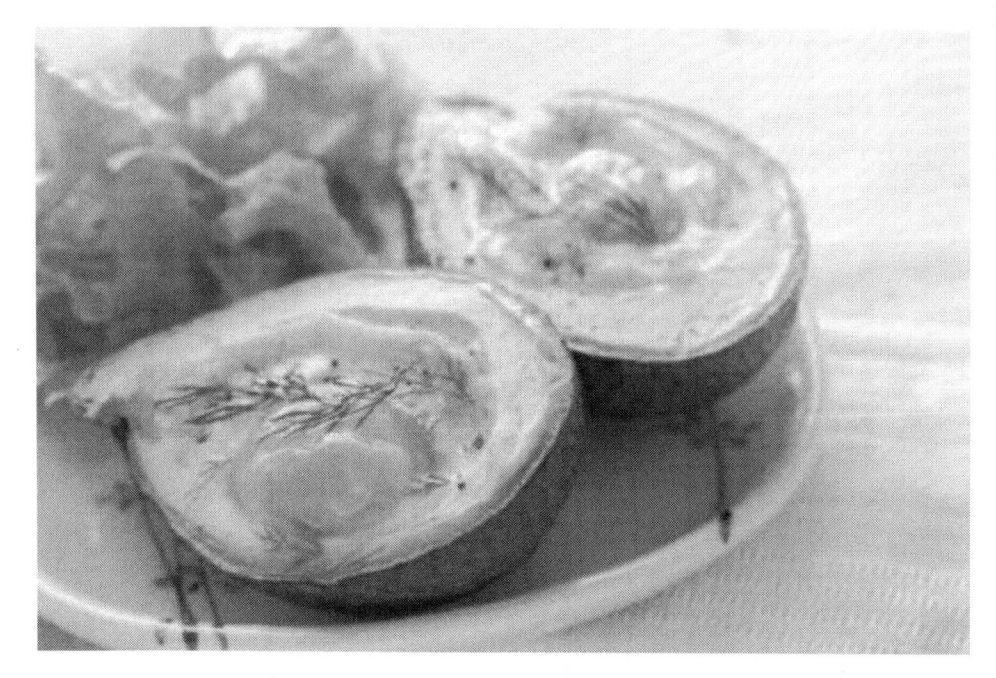

Nutrition Facts Per Serving

Calories	Fats	Proteins	Carbohydrates
334	28	16	4.6

Ingredients

Serves	1	2	3	4	5	6	7	8
Tuna, canned, drained, ounces	1	2	3	4	5	6	7	8
Avocado, pitted	½	1	1 ½	2	2 ½	3	3 ½	4
Egg, pasteurized	1	2	3	4	5	6	7	8
Avocado oil, tablespoon	1	2	3	4	5	6	7	8
Salt, by taste								
Black pepper, by taste								

Instructions

1. Switch on the oven, then set it to 425 degrees F, and let it preheat.
2. In the meantime, enlarge the hollow of the avocado by scooping some flesh from the center of the avocado half, and then place the tuna in it.
3. Crack the egg into the avocado and then bake for 10 minutes or more until the egg has cooked.
4. When done, sprinkle salt and black pepper over the egg, drizzle with oil, and then serve.

Stuffed Zucchini Boats

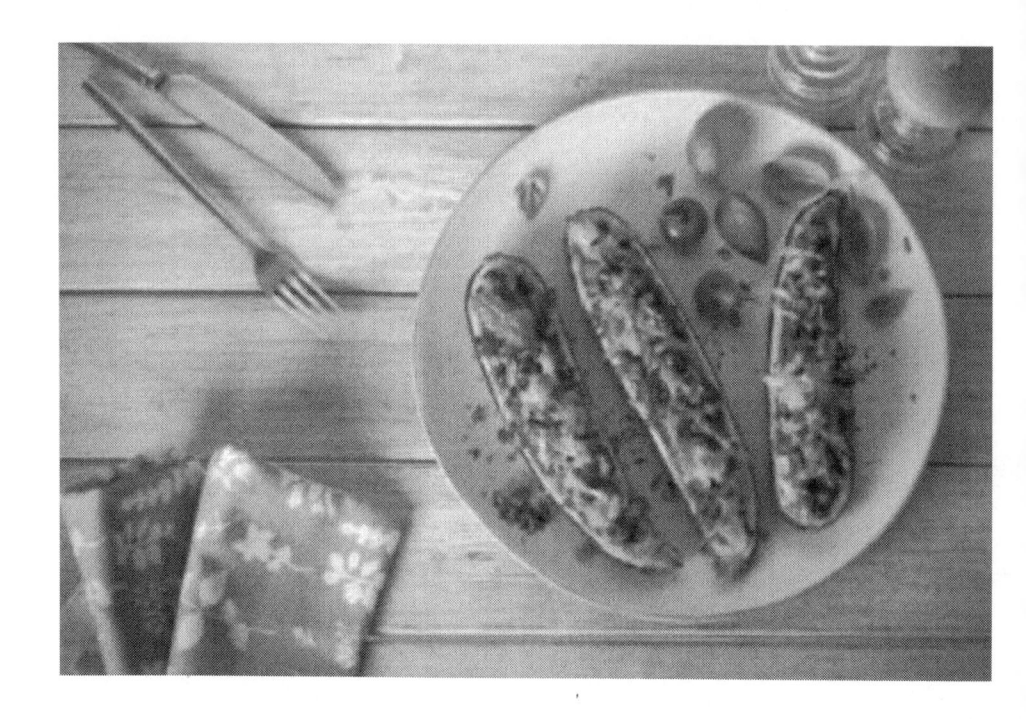

Nutrition Facts Per Serving

Calories	Fats	Proteins	Carbohydrates
888	70.1	53.3	11.1

Ingredients

Serves	1	2	3	4	5	6	7	8
Zucchini, medium	1	2	3	4	5	6	7	8
Ground beef, grass-fed, ounces	5	10	15	20	25	30	35	40
Tomato sauce, cup	1/3	2/3	1	1 1/3	1 2/3	2	2 1/3	2 2/3
Cheddar cheese, grated, cup	1/2	1	1 1/2	2	2 1/2	3	3 1/2	4
Avocado oil, tablespoon	2	4	6	8	10	12	14	16
Salt, teaspoon	1	2	3	4	5	6	7	8
Italian seasoning, teaspoon	1/2	1	1 1/2	2	2 1/2	3	3 1/2	4

Instructions

1. Switch on the oven, then set it to 400 degrees F, and let it preheat.
2. In the meantime, halve the zucchini lengthwise, and then make some space along its center by using a spoon.
3. Place the zucchini halves cut-side up on a foil-lined baking sheet and then drizzle with 1 tablespoon oil.
4. Sprinkle ½ teaspoon salt over the zucchini and then bake for 15 minutes or more until roasted and softened.
5. While the zucchini bakes, place the oil in a medium skillet pan over medium heat and when hot, add the beef and cook for 10 minutes or more until golden brown.
6. Season the beef with Italian seasoning and remaining salt, cook for 1 minute, and then remove the pan from heat.
7. Add 1/3 cup of cheese in the pan along with tomato sauce and then stir until well mixed.
8. When the zucchini has baked, pat it dry, stuff the zucchini halves with the beef mixture, and then sprinkle cheese on top.
9. Return the zucchini halves into the oven and then bake for 5 minutes until the cheese melts.
10. Serve immediately.

Lettuce Wraps

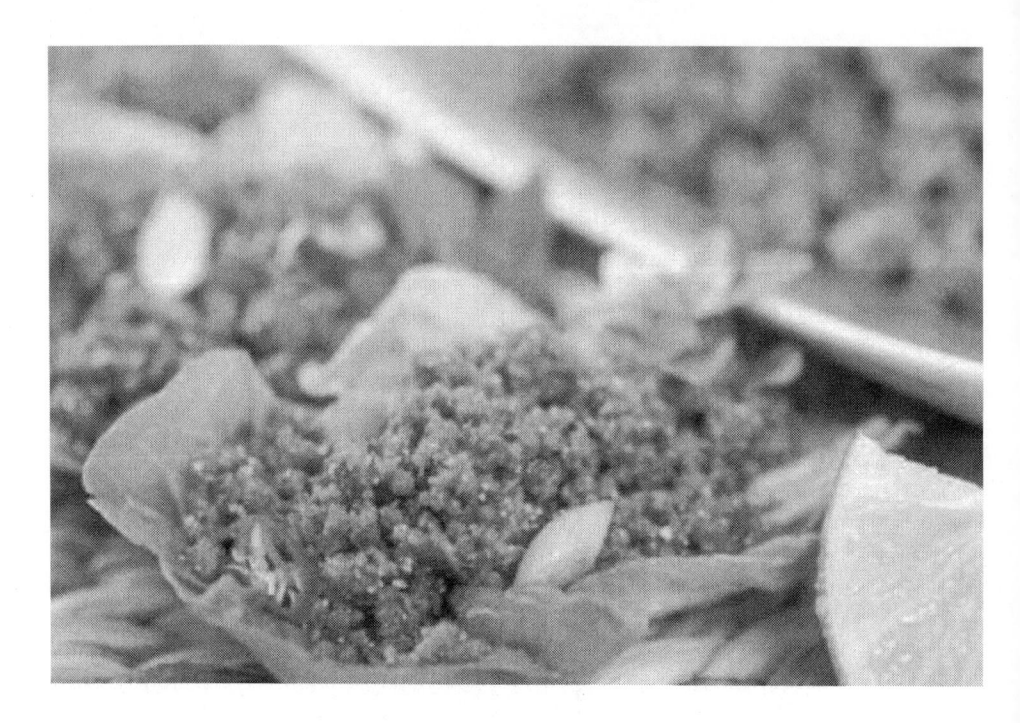

Nutrition Facts Per Serving

Calories	Fats	Proteins	Carbohydrates
297	25.1	17.1	0.7

Ingredients

Serves	1	2	3	4	5	6	7	8
Ground beef, grass-fed, ounces	2	4	6	8	10	12	14	16
Lettuce leaf, large	1	2	3	4	5	6	7	8
Sesame oil, tablespoon	1	2	3	4	5	6	7	8
Soy sauce, tablespoon	1	2	3	4	5	6	7	8
Cheddar cheese, grated, tablespoon	1	2	3	4	5	6	7	8
Salt, teaspoon	¼	½	¾	1	1 ¼	1 ½	1 ¾	2
Black pepper, teaspoon	¼	½	¾	1	1 ¼	1 ½	1 ¾	2

Instructions

1. Place a medium skillet pan over medium heat; and when hot, add the beef and then cook it for 10 minutes or more until golden brown and cooked.
2. In the meantime, pour the oil in a small bowl, add soy sauce, salt, and black pepper and stir until mixed.
3. Pour the sauce over the beef, stir until mixed, and then cook for 3 minutes until the sauce has evaporated.
4. Spoon the beef mixture over the leaf, sprinkle cheese on it, fold it like a wrap, and then serve.

Creamy Broccoli Salad

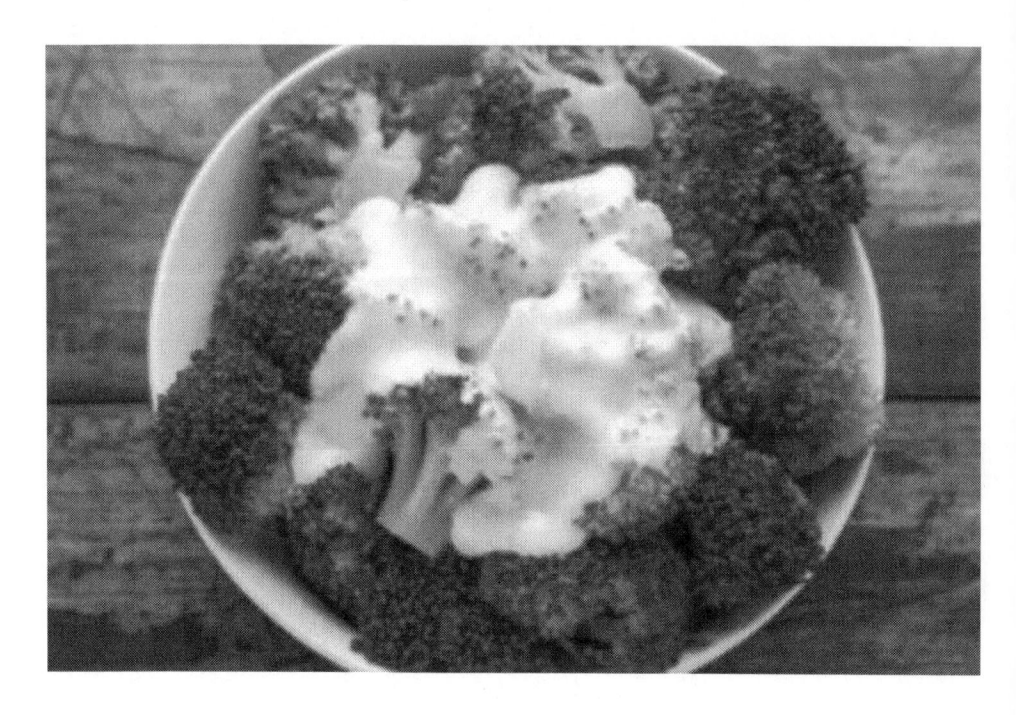

Nutrition Facts Per Serving

Calories	Fats	Proteins	Carbohydrates
328	31	8.2	4.1

Ingredients

Serves	1	2	3	4	5	6	7	8
Chopped broccoli florets, cup	½	1	1 ½	2	2 ½	3	3 ½	4
Heavy cream, full-fat, tablespoon	2	4	6	8	10	12	14	16
Bacon slice	2	4	6	8	10	12	14	16
Garlic powder, teaspoon	1/3	2/3	1	1 1/3	1 2/3	2	2 1/3	2 2/3
Dried parsley, teaspoon	1/8	1/4	1/3	½	2/3	¾	1	1 1/8
Salt, teaspoon	1/8	1/4	1/3	½	2/3	¾	1	1 1/8

Instructions

1. Place a medium frying pan over medium heat and when hot, place bacon slices, and then cook for 2 to 3 minutes per side until cooked and tender-crisp.
2. Transfer the bacon to a cutting board, let it cool for 5 minutes, and then chop it.
3. Place the cream in a salad bowl, add parsley and garlic, and then whisk until smooth.
4. Add the broccoli, fold it until coated, and then top with cheese and bacon. Lastly, serve.

Tuna Cakes

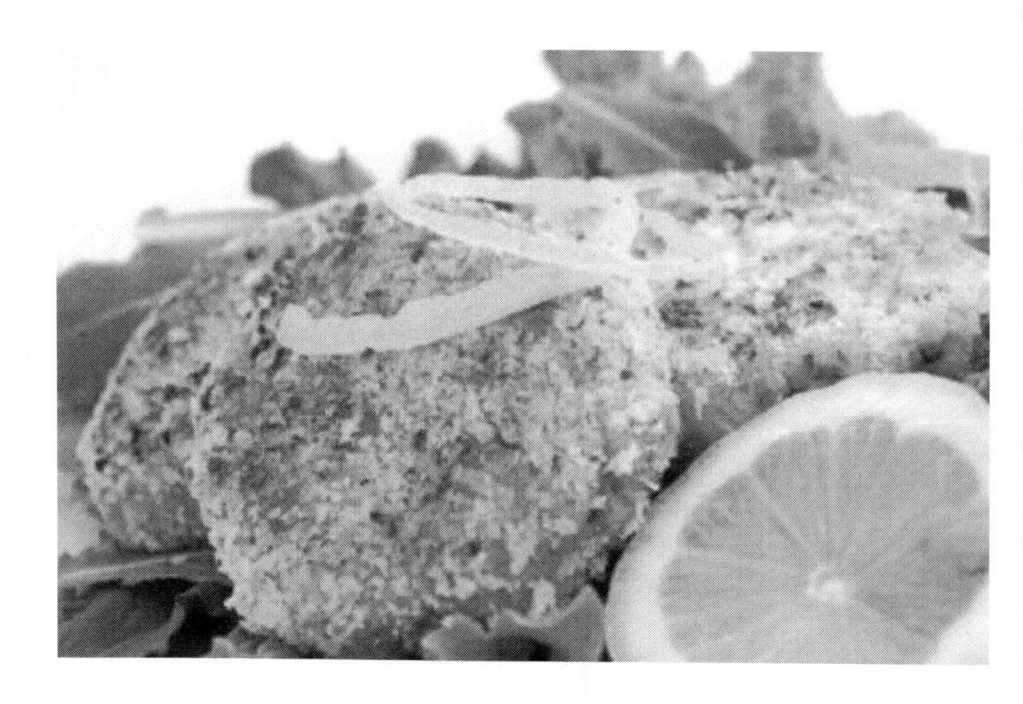

Nutrition Facts Per Serving

Calories	Fats	Proteins	Carbohydrates
425	29.3	39.3	1.1

Ingredients

Serves	1	2	3	4	5	6	7	8
Tuna, canned, drained, ounces	5	10	15	20	25	30	35	40
Spring onion, medium	1	2	3	4	5	6	7	8
Mustard paste, tablespoon	1	2	3	4	5	6	7	8
Garlic powder, teaspoon	1	2	3	4	5	6	7	8
Avocado oil, tablespoon	2	4	6	8	10	12	14	16
Salt, by taste	¼	½	¾	2	2 ¼	2 ½	2 ¾	3
Black pepper, by taste	¼	½	¾	2	2 ¼	2 ½	2 ¾	3

Instructions

1. Chop the onion, place it in a medium bowl, add the tuna, and then crumble it.
2. Add the remaining ingredients, except for the oil, stir until well combined, and then shape the mixture into two patties.
3. Place the oil in a medium skillet pan over medium heat and when hot, add patties to the pan and then cook for 4 to 5 minutes per side until golden brown.
4. Serve swiftly.

Spinach Stuffed Zucchini

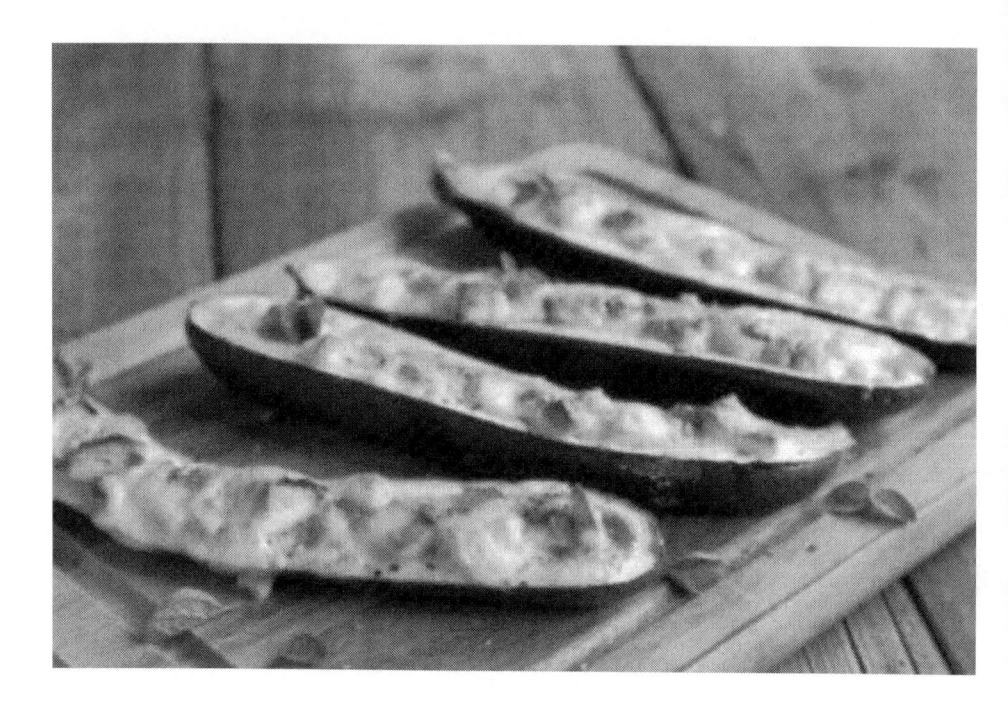

Nutrition Facts Per Serving

Calories	Fats	Proteins	Carbohydrates
529	48.2	15.9	7.9

Ingredients

Serves	1	2	3	4	5	6	7	8
Zucchini, medium	1	2	3	4	5	6	7	8
Spinach, cup	2/3	1 1/3	2	2 2/3	3 1/3	4	4 2/3	5 1/3
Heavy cream, full-fat, tablespoon	3	6	9	12	15	18	21	24
Parmesan cheese, grated, full-fat, tablespoon	2	4	6	8	10	12	14	16
Bacon slice	2	4	6	8	10	12	14	16
Avocado oil, tablespoon	1½	3	4½	6	7½	9	10½	12
Salt, teaspoon	¾	1½	2¼	3	3¾	4½	5¼	6

Instructions

1. Switch on the oven, then set it to 350 degrees F, and let it preheat.
2. In the meantime, place ½ tablespoon oil in a medium skillet pan, place it over medium heat, and when hot, add the spinach.
3. Stir until the spinach is coated in oil and then cook for 5 minutes or more until tender, and all the moisture in the pan has evaporated.
4. When done, stir in ¼ teaspoon salt, add cream and 1 tablespoon cheese, stir until cheese melts, and then remove the pan from the heat.
5. While the spinach cooks, halve the zucchini lengthwise and then make some space along its center using a spoon.
6. Place zucchini halves cut-side up on a foil-lined baking sheet and then drizzle with the remaining oil.
7. Sprinkle ½ teaspoon salt over the zucchini and then bake for 10 minutes until tender.
8. Then pat dry the zucchini halves, stuff them with the spinach mixture, sprinkle the remaining cheese on top and then broil for 3 minutes until cheese has melted and turned golden brown.
9. Serve immediately.

Cider Chicken Thighs

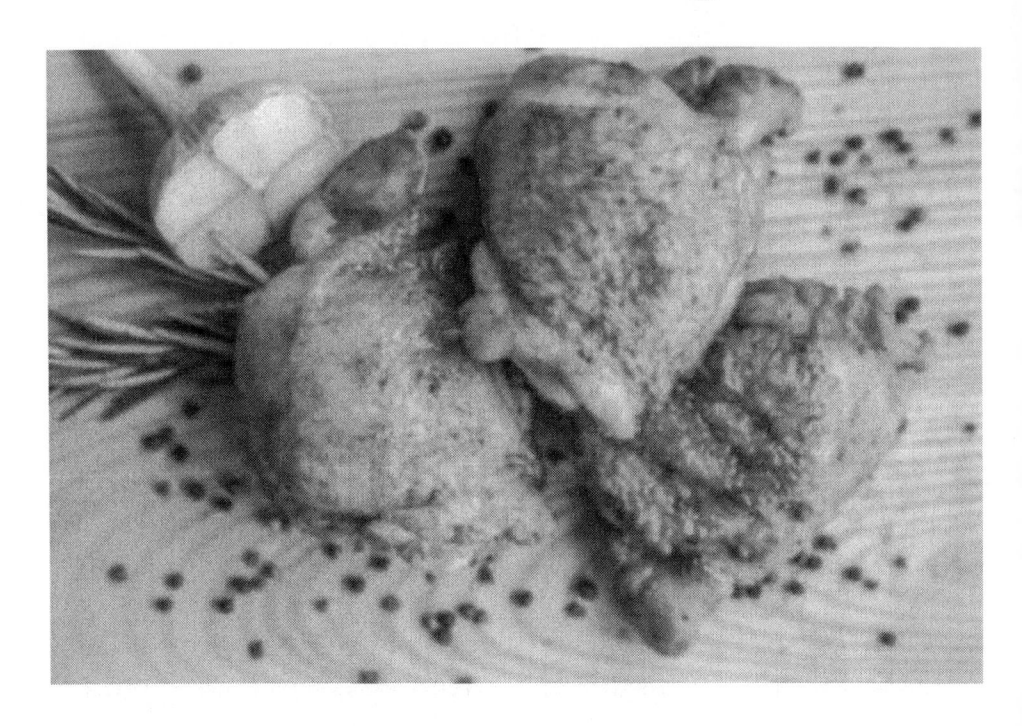

Nutrition Facts Per Serving

Calories	Fats	Proteins	Carbohydrates
552	37.4	53.8	0

Ingredients

Serves	1	2	3	4	5	6	7	8
Chicken thighs, large, pasteurized	2	4	6	8	10	12	14	16
Apple cider vinegar, cup	¼	½	¾	1	1¼	1½	1¾	2
Liquid stevia, teaspoon	1	2	3	4	5	6	7	8
Avocado oil, tablespoon	2	4	6	8	10	12	14	16
Salt, teaspoon	1	2	3	4	5	6	7	8
Black pepper, teaspoon	1	2	3	4	5	6	7	8

Instructions

1. Switch on the oven, set it to 450 degrees F, and let it preheat.
2. Take a shallow dish, place the chicken in it, season with salt and black pepper, drizzle with oil, and then rub generously.
3. Arrange the chicken on a baking sheet and then bake for 8 minutes per side until thoroughly cooked.
4. In the meantime, pour the vinegar in a small saucepan, add stevia, place the pan over medium heat, and bring it to a boil.
5. When the vinegar mixture begins to boil, switch the heat to the low level and then simmer for 4 to 5 minutes until the sauce has reduced by half.
6. When the chicken has cooked, brush it on all sides with the vinegar sauce, then place the chicken under broiler and cook it for 2 minutes per side until golden brown.
7. Serve immediately.

Bacon Wrapped Asparagus

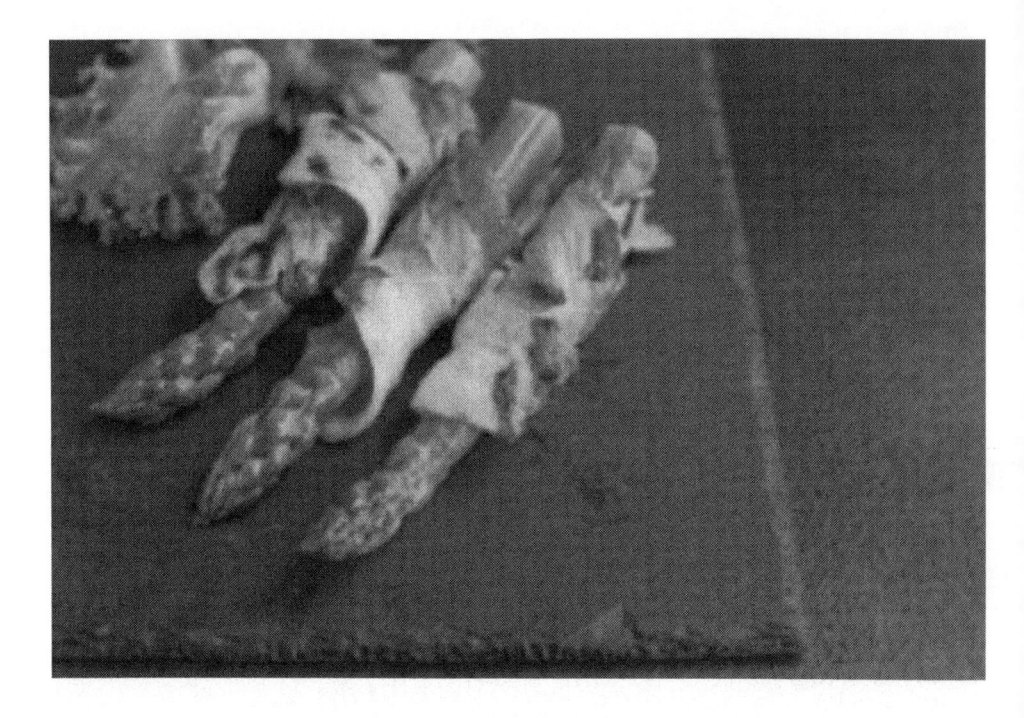

Nutrition Facts Per Serving

Calories	Fats	Proteins	Carbohydrates
220	20	6	3

Ingredients

Serves	1	2	3	4	5	6	7	8
Asparagus stalks, trimmed	4	8	12	16	20	24	28	32
Bacon slice, pasteurized	2	4	6	8	10	12	14	16
Avocado oil, teaspoon	1	2	3	4	5	6	7	8
Garlic salt, to taste								
Ground black pepper, to taste								

Instructions

1. Switch on the oven, set it to 400 degrees F, and let it preheat.
2. Prepare the asparagus and for this, drizzle it with oil, and then season with garlic salt and black pepper.
3. Cut out lengthwise strips from the bacon slices and then wrap each bacon strip on a piece of asparagus in striped patterns.
4. Take a sheet pan, place it on a wire rack, arrange the bacon wrapped asparagus, and then bake for 10 minutes per side until the bacon becomes crisp.
5. Then switch on the broiler and then continue cooking for 2 minutes.
6. Serve swiftly.

Beef Stuffed Avocado

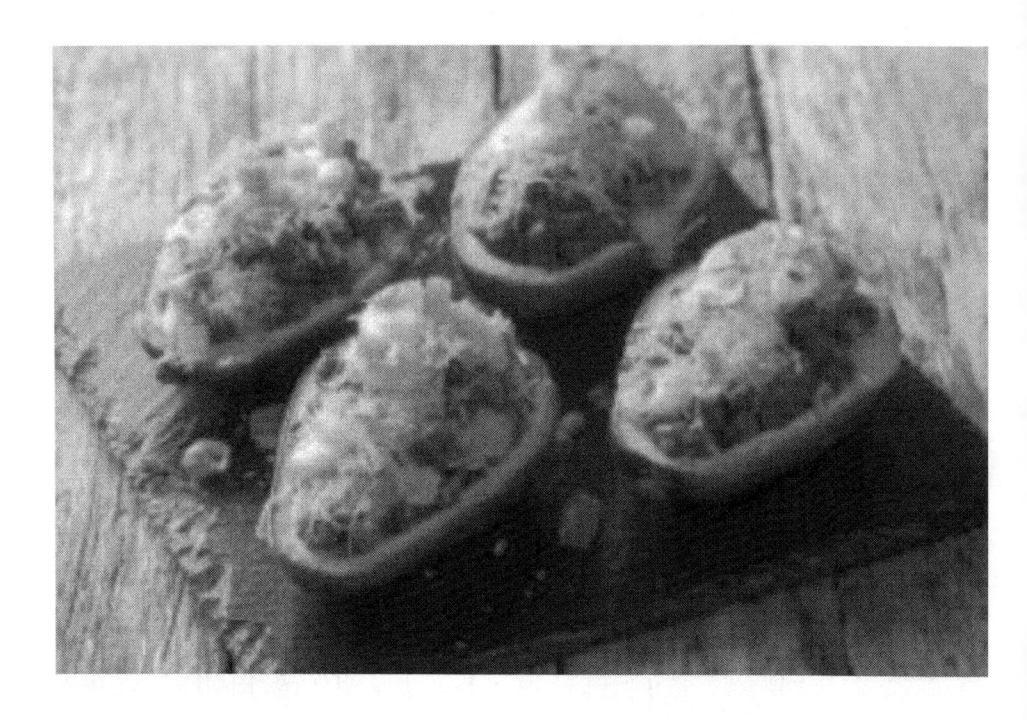

Nutrition Facts Per Serving

Calories	Fats	Proteins	Carbohydrates
398	31	24.9	5

Ingredients

Serves	1	2	3	4	5	6	7	8
Ground beef, grass-fed, ounces	3	6	9	12	15	18	21	24
Avocado, large	½	1	1½	2	2½	3	3½	4
Avocado oil, teaspoon	1	2	3	4	5	6	7	8
Garlic powder	½	1	1½	2	2½	3	3½	4
Cheddar cheese, grated, full-fat, tablespoon	1	2	3	4	5	6	7	8
Salt, by taste	1/3	2/3	1	1 1/3	1 2/3	2	2 1/3	2 2/3
Black pepper, by taste	1/3	2/3	1	1 1/3	1 2/3	2	2 1/3	2 2/3

Instructions

1. Place the oil in a medium skillet pan over medium heat and when hot, add beef, season with salt, and cook it for 5 minutes or until nicely brown.
2. Remove the pit from the avocado, scoop out some more flesh from it to make space for the beef, and then stuff the avocado half with beef.
3. Sprinkle the cheese over the beef, place it under the broiler, and then bake it for 2 minutes or more until the cheese melts.
4. Serve punctually.

Salmon Patties

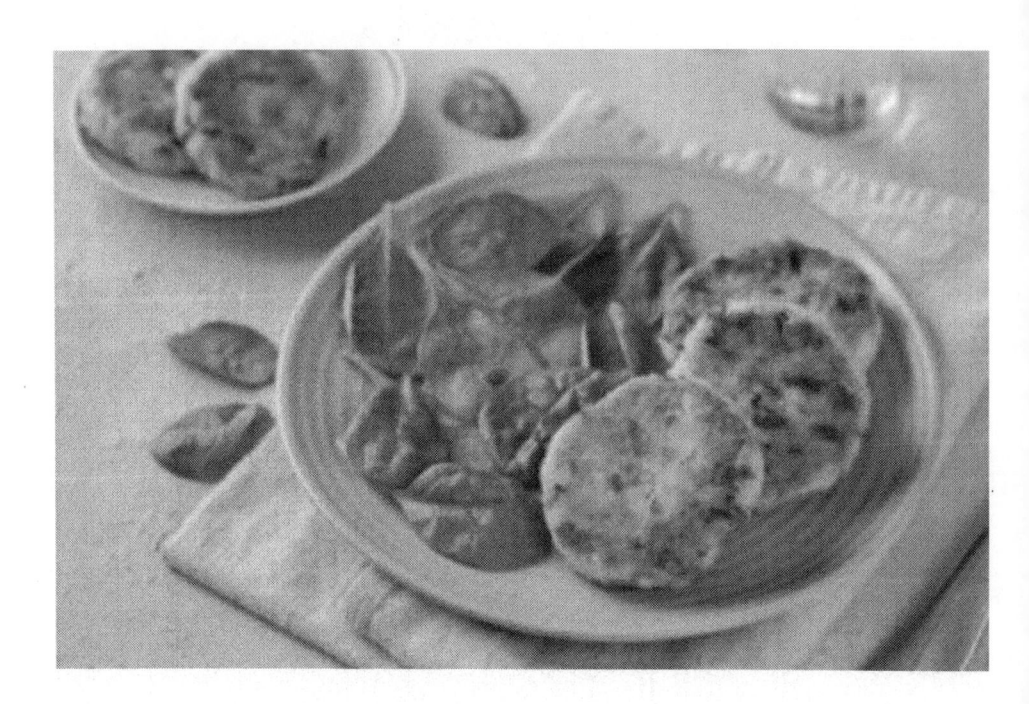

Nutrition Facts Per Serving

Calories	Fats	Proteins	Carbohydrates
606	49.8	37.9	1.5

Ingredients

Serves	1	2	3	4	5	6	7	8
Salmon, canned, drained	4	8	12	16	20	24	28	32
Egg, pasteurized	1	2	3	4	5	6	7	8
Chopped cilantro, tablespoon	1	2	3	4	5	6	7	8
Avocado oil, tablespoon	1	2	3	4	5	6	7	8
Mayonnaise, full-fat, tablespoon	2	4	6	8	10	12	14	16
Salt, by taste	¼	½	¾	1	1¼	1½	1¾	2
Black pepper, by taste	¼	½	¾	1	1¼	1½	1¾	2

Instructions

1. Place the salmon in a medium bowl and then add the remaining ingredients except for the oil.
2. Stir until combined and then shape the mixture into two evenly size patties.
3. Place the oil in a medium skillet pan over medium heat. Next and when hot, add the patties and then cook for 4 to 5 minutes per side until golden brown.
4. Serve immediately.

Cheesy Zoodles

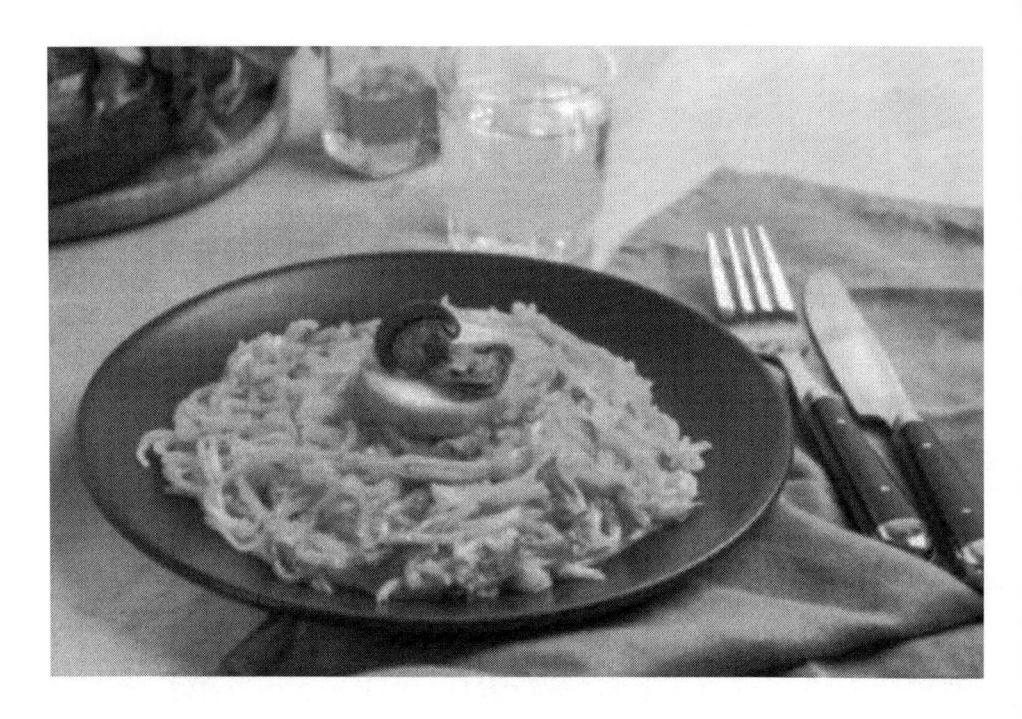

Nutrition Facts Per Serving

Calories	Fats	Proteins	Carbohydrates
740	67.4	22.2	11.1

Ingredients

Serves	1	2	3	4	5	6	7	8
Zucchini, spiralized into noodles	1	2	3	4	5	6	7	8
Parmesan cheese, grated, full-fat, tablespoon	2	4	6	8	10	12	14	16
Cream cheese, softened, full-fat, tablespoon	2	4	6	8	10	12	14	16
Bacon slice, chopped	4	8	12	16	20	24	28	32
Avocado oil, tablespoon	1	2	3	4	5	6	7	8
Salt, by taste								
Black pepper, by taste								

Instructions

1. Place a skillet pan over medium heat and when hot, add the chopped bacon and then cook it for 4 to 5 minutes until tender and crisp.
2. Transfer the bacon to a bowl, add oil in it and when hot, add the zucchini noodles, and then toss until coated in oil.
3. Cook the noodles for 4 to 5 minutes until tender and crispy, and then push them to one side of the pan. Next, add the cream cheese to the empty side of the pan and let it melt.
4. When the cream cheese has melted, stir the noodles in it, add the bacon, season with salt and black pepper, sprinkle with cheese, and stir until the cheese melts.
5. Serve punctually.

Taco Radish Wedges

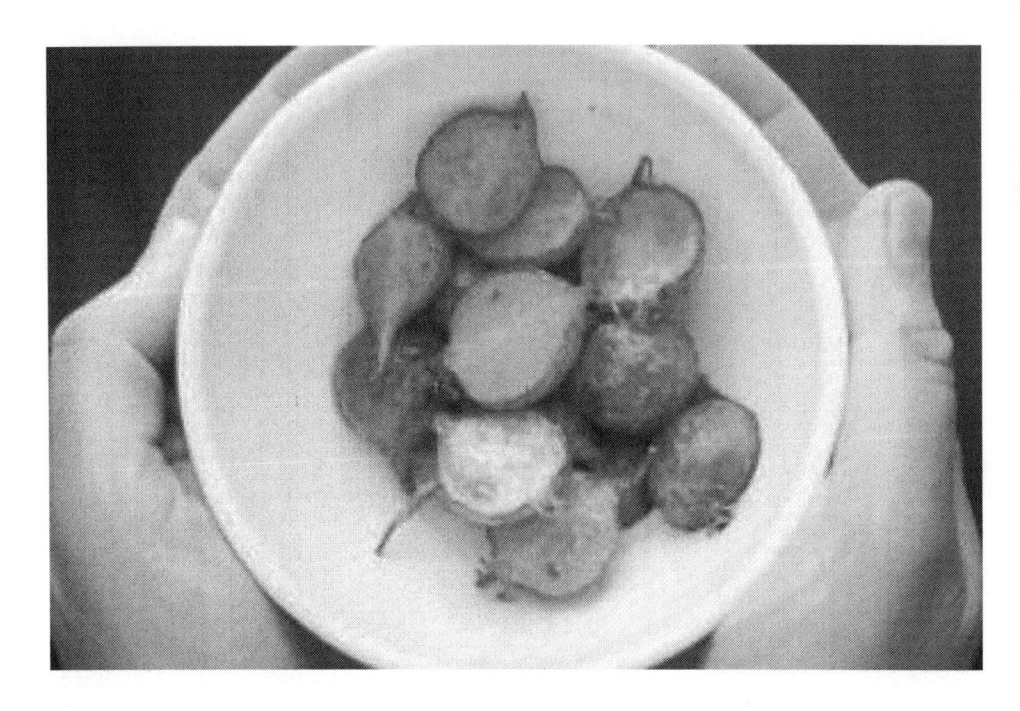

Nutrition Facts Per Serving

Calories	Fats	Proteins	Carbohydrates
419	40.5	8.4	5.2

Ingredients

Serves	1	2	3	4	5	6	7	8
Radish, large, bunch	1	2	3	4	5	6	7	8
Bacon slice, chopped	2	4	6	8	10	12	14	16
Taco seasoning, teaspoon	2	4	6	8	10	12	14	16
Avocado oil, tablespoon	1	2	3	4	5	6	7	8
Cream cheese, softened, full-fat, tablespoon	2	4	6	8	10	12	14	16

Instructions

1. Switch on the oven, set it to 400 degrees F, and let it preheat.
2. In the meantime, cut the radish into wedges and then place them in a bowl.
3. Drizzle oil over the radish chunks, sprinkle with taco seasoning, and then toss until coated.
4. Spread the radish wedges in a single layer over the foil-lined baking sheet and then bake 40 minutes until crisp, turning halfway.
5. In the meantime, place a skillet pan over medium heat; when hot, add chopped bacon and then cook it for 3 to 5 minutes until tender-crisp. Finally, set aside until required.
6. When the radish wedges have baked, top them with bacon and cream cheese before serving.

Sweet and Spicy Brussel Sprouts

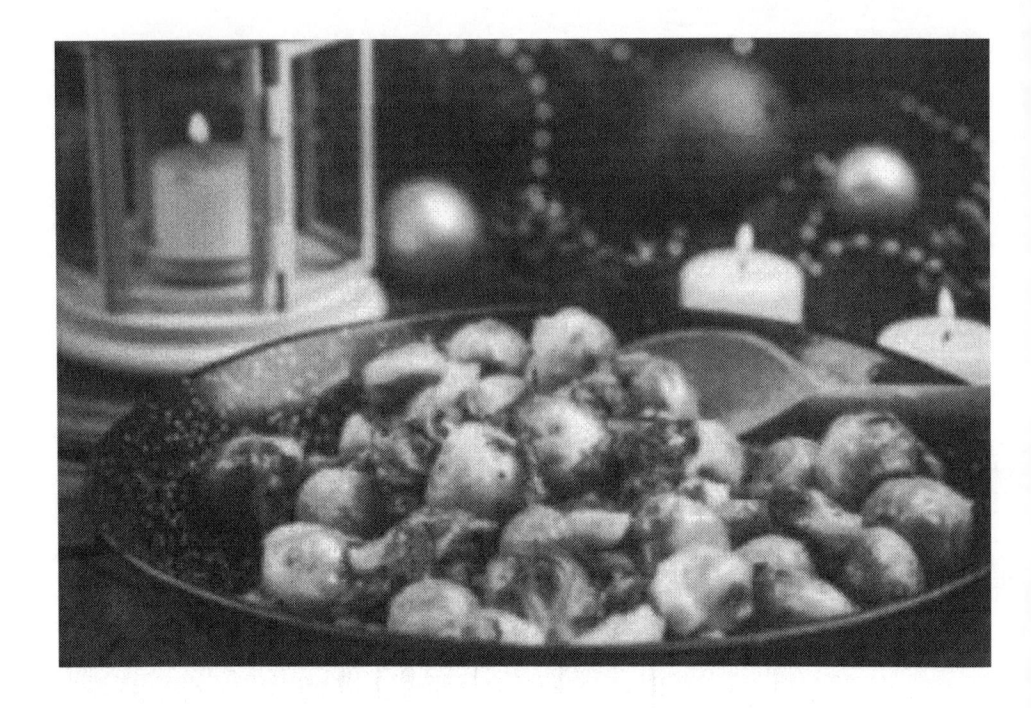

Nutrition Facts Per Serving

Calories	Fats	Proteins	Carbohydrates
489	47.3	9.8	6.1

Ingredients

Serves	1	2	3	4	5	6	7	8
Brussel Sprouts, halved, ounces	3	6	9	12	15	18	21	24
Bacon slice, chopped	2	4	6	8	10	12	14	16
Soy sauce, tablespoon	1 ½	3	4 ½	6	7 ½	9	10 ½	12
Liquid stevia, tablespoon	¾	1 ½	2 ¼	3	3 ¾	4 ½	5 ¼	6
Avocado oil, tablespoon	2	4	6	8	10	12	14	16
Salt, teaspoon	1/3	2/3	1	1 1/3	1 2/3	2	2 1/3	2 2/3

Instructions

1. Place a skillet pan over medium heat; and when hot, add chopped bacon and then cook it for 4 to 5 minutes until tender and crisp.
2. Transfer the bacon to a bowl, add oil to it, and when hot, add the Brussel sprouts and cook for 10 to 12 minutes until golden brown on all sides and almost cooked.
3. In the meantime, pour soy sauce in a small bowl, add stevia, and then stir until mixed.
4. When the Brussel sprouts have cooked, season with salt, drizzle with the soy sauce mixture, toss until coated, and cook for 2 minutes until thoroughly cooked.
5. Garnish the Brussel sprouts with bacon and then serve.

Paprika Chicken

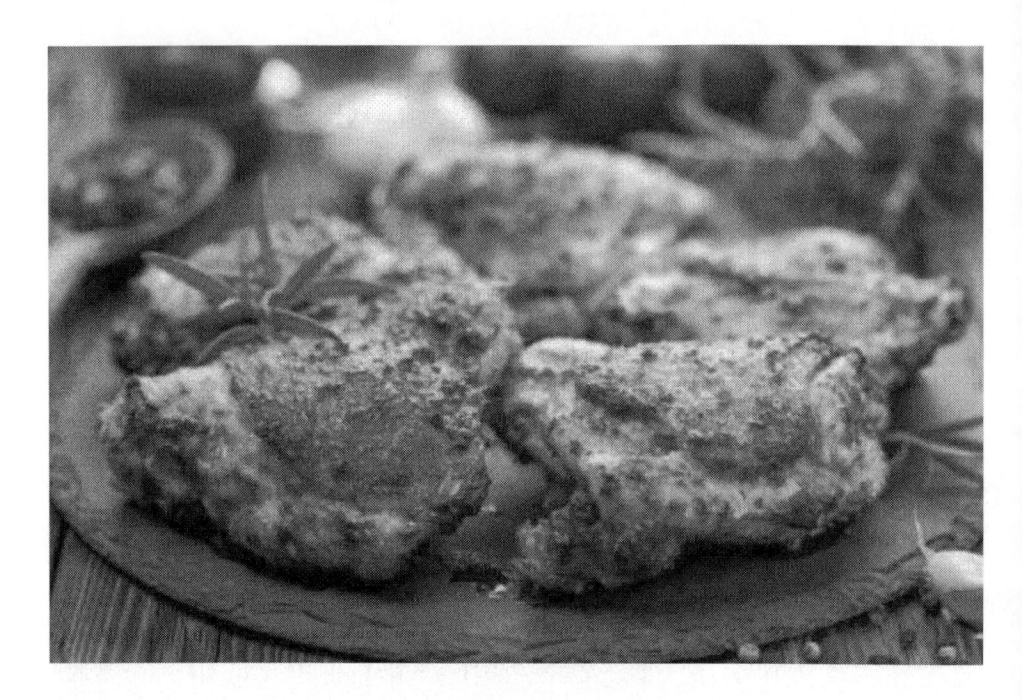

Nutrition Facts Per Serving

Calories	Fats	Proteins	Carbohydrates
552	37.4	53.8	0

Ingredients

Serves	1	2	3	4	5	6	7	8
Chicken thighs, large, pasteurized	2	4	6	8	10	12	14	16
Hot paprika, teaspoon	1	2	3	4	5	6	7	8
Smoked paprika, teaspoon	½	1	1½	2	2½	3	3½	4
Garlic powder, teaspoon	½	1	1½	2	2½	3	3½	4
Avocado oil, tablespoon	2	4	6	8	10	12	14	16
Salt, teaspoon	1	2	3	4	5	6	7	8

Instructions

1. Switch on the oven, set it to 325 degrees F, and let it preheat.
2. In the meantime, place the hot and smoked paprika in a small bowl, add garlic powder, salt, and avocado oil, and then stir until combined.
3. Brush this mixture generously on all sides of the chicken, arrange on a foil-lined baking sheet, and then bake for 12 minutes per side until cooked and tender.
4. Serve right away.

Egg and Spinach Salad

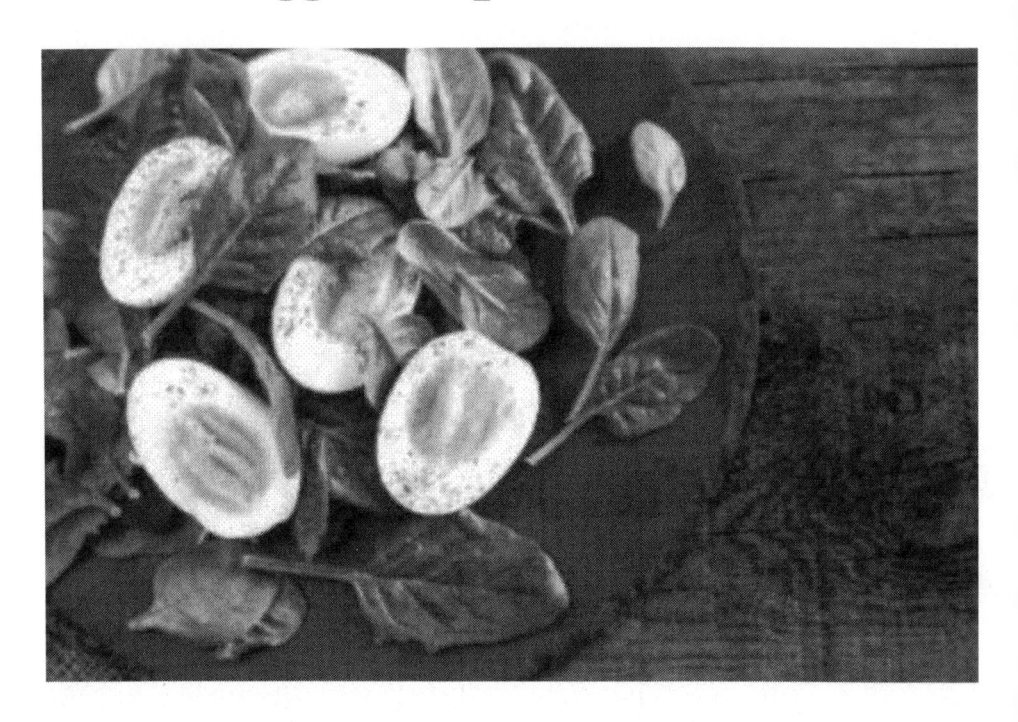

Nutrition Facts Per Serving

Calories	Fats	Proteins	Carbohydrates
712	65	28.5	3.6

Ingredients

Serves	1	2	3	4	5	6	7	8
Spinach, fresh, ounces	2	4	6	8	10	12	14	16
Bacon slice, chopped	4	8	12	16	20	24	28	32
Eggs, pasteurized, boiled	2	4	6	8	10	12	14	16
Avocado oil, tablespoon	1	2	3	4	5	6	7	8
Salt, by taste								
Black pepper, by taste								

Instructions

1. Place a skillet pan over medium heat until hot. Next, add chopped bacon and then cook it for 4 to 5 minutes until tender-crisp.
2. Transfer the bacon to a bowl, add spinach, drizzle with oil and then toss until coated.
3. Peel the boiled eggs, cut them into slices, add them to the salad bowl, and then sprinkle with salt and black pepper.
4. Serve ASAP.

Cheesy Cauliflower Soup

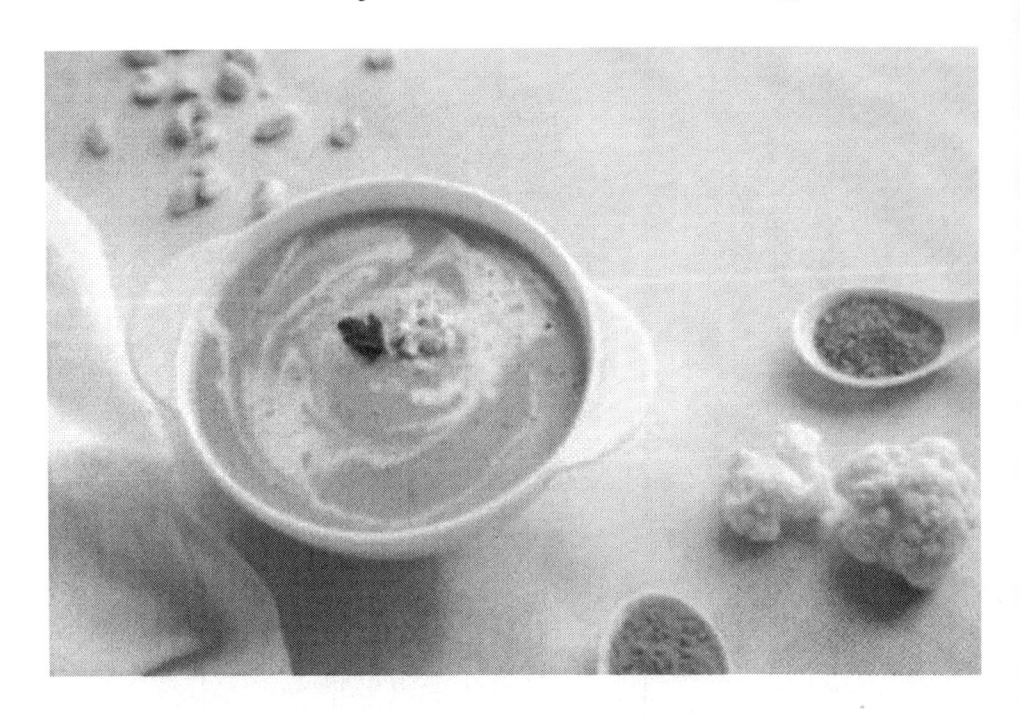

Nutrition Facts Per Serving

Calories	Fats	Proteins	Carbohydrates
591	51.9	23.6	7.4

Ingredients

Serves	1	2	3	4	5	6	7	8
Chopped cauliflower, ounces	4	8	12	16	20	24	28	32
Bacon slice, chopped	2	4	6	8	10	12	14	16
Heavy cream, full-fat, tablespoon	2	4	6	8	10	12	14	16
Chicken broth, pasteurized, cup	1 1/2	3	4 1/2	6	7 1/2	9	10 1/2	12
Parmesan cheese, grated, full-fat, tablespoon	2	4	6	8	10	12	14	16
Salt, teaspoon	1/3	2/3	1	1 1/3	1 2/3	2	2 1/3	2 2/3
Black pepper, teaspoon	1/3	2/3	1	1 1/3	1 2/3	2	2 1/3	2 2/3

Instructions

1. Place a medium pot over medium heat and when hot, add the chopped bacon and then cook it for 4 to 5 minutes until tender-crisp.
2. Transfer the bacon to a bowl, add oil into the pot, and then add the cauliflower in it.
3. Season with salt and black pepper, pour in the broth and then bring the soup to a boil.
4. Switch the heat to medium-low level and then simmer for 7 to 10 minutes until the cauliflower turns tender, covering the pot with its lid.
5. When done, remove the pot from heat, and then puree the soup by using an immersion blender.
6. Add the cream and cheese into the soup, stir until cheese melts, and then taste to adjust the seasoning.
7. Garnish the soup with bacon, drizzle with avocado oil, and then serve.

Spinach Salad with Feta Dressing

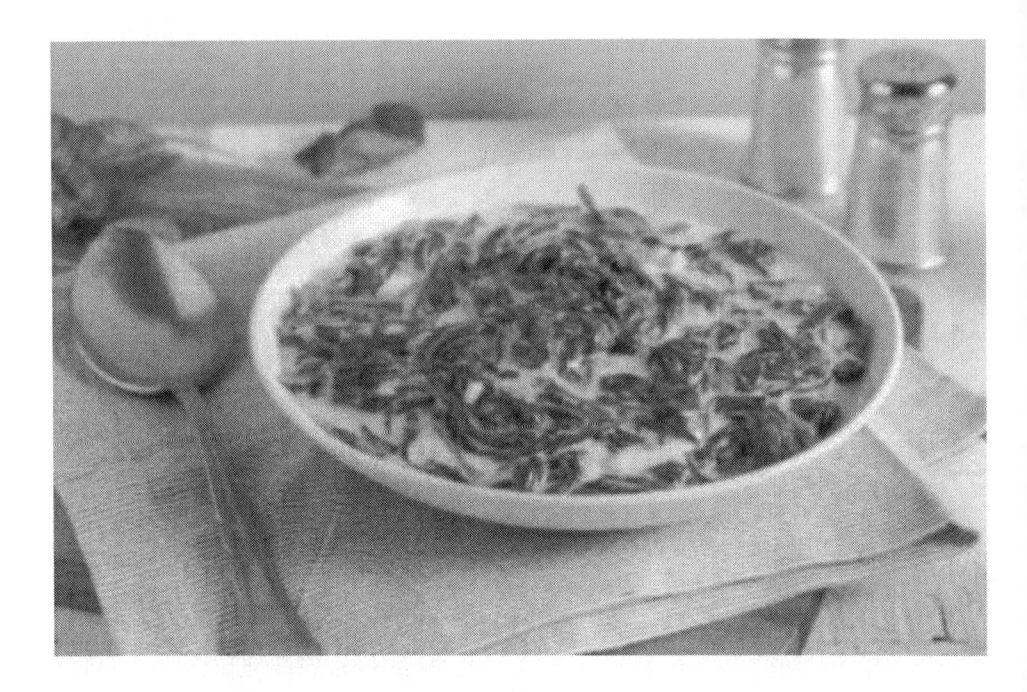

Nutrition Facts Per Serving

Calories	Fats	Proteins	Carbohydrates
479	44.7	14.4	4.8

Ingredients

Serves	1	2	3	4	5	6	7	8
Spinach, fresh, ounces	4	8	12	16	20	24	28	32
Avocado oil, tablespoon	2	4	6	8	10	12	14	16
Feta cheese, full-fat, crumbled	3	6	9	12	15	18	21	24
Apple cider vinegar, tablespoon	2	4	6	8	10	12	14	16
Salt, by taste								
Black pepper, by taste								

Instructions

1. Take a microwave-oven proof bowl, place cheese in it, and then microwave it for 30 to 60 seconds until slightly melted.
2. Then stir in vinegar immediately and set aside until required.
3. Place the spinach in a salad, season with salt and black pepper, drizzle with oil, and then toss until mixed.
4. Top the spinach with feta cheese and then serve.

Lettuce and Avocado Rolls

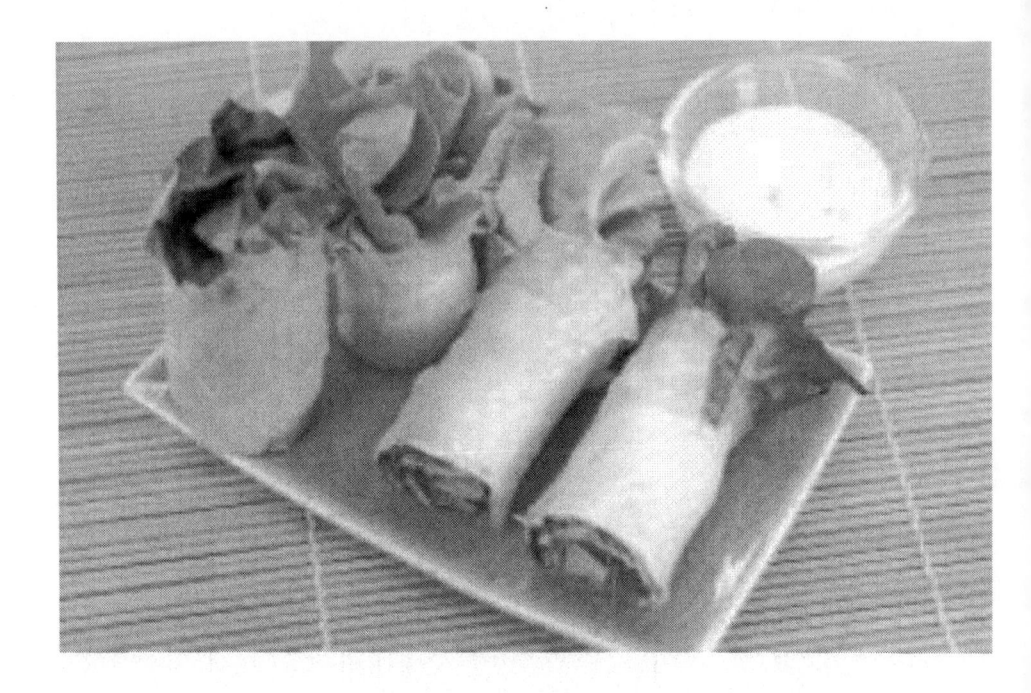

Nutrition Facts Per Serving

Calories	Fats	Proteins	Carbohydrates
489	46.2	12.2	6.1

Ingredients

Serves	1	2	3	4	5	6	7	8
Lettuce leaf, large	1	2	3	4	5	6	7	8
Avocado, pitted, sliced	½	1	1½	2	2½	3	3½	4
Butter, unsalted, tablespoon	1	2	3	4	5	6	7	8
Cheddar cheese, grated, full-fat, tablespoon	2	4	6	8	10	12	14	16
Lime juice, teaspoon	1	2	3	4	5	6	7	8

Instructions

1. Place a medium pot over medium heat and when hot, add the bacon slices and then cook it for 4 to 5 minutes until tender-crisp.
2. Pat dry the lettuce leaf, spread butter on top, and then arrange bacon slices on it.
3. Cut the avocado into slices, place them on one side of the leaf, and then sprinkle with cheese and roll.
4. Serve swiftly.

Garlic Zoodles

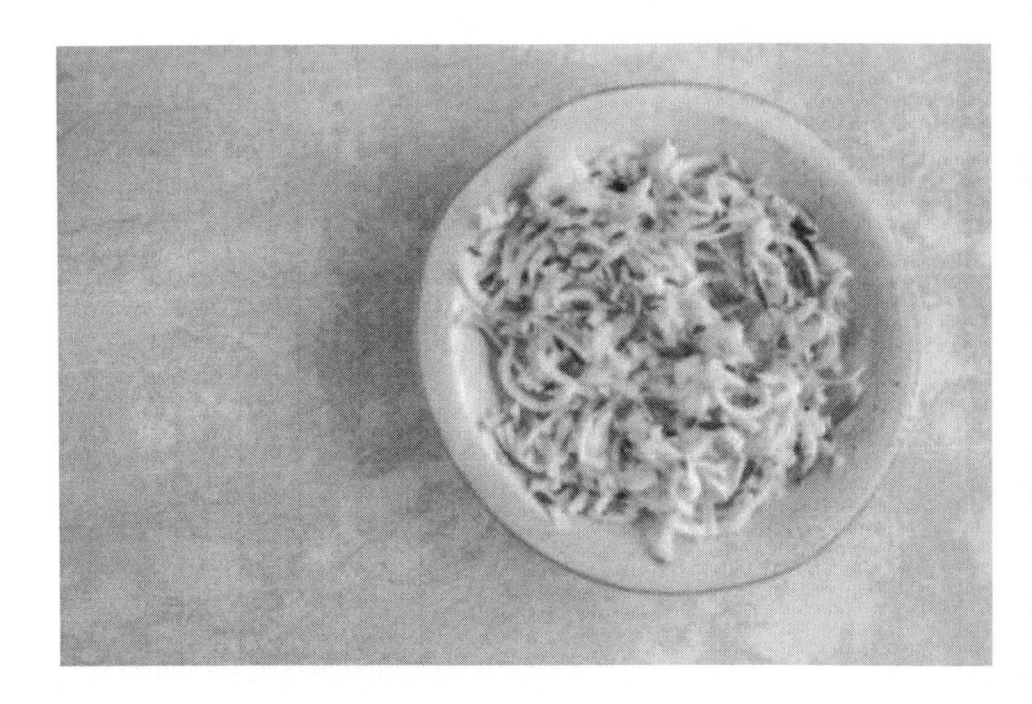

Nutrition Facts Per Serving

Calories	Fats	Proteins	Carbohydrates
499	50.5	3.7	7.5

Ingredients

Serves	1	2	3	4	5	6	7	8
Zucchini, large, spiralized into noodles	1	2	3	4	5	6	7	8
Lime juice, teaspoon	2	4	6	8	10	12	14	16
Butter, unsalted, tablespoon	2	4	6	8	10	12	14	16
Avocado oil, tablespoon	2	4	6	8	10	12	14	16
Sriracha sauce, tablespoon	1	2	3	4	5	6	7	8
Salt, by taste								
Black pepper, by taste								

Instructions

1. Place oil and butter in a medium skillet pan; and when the butter melts, add lime juice and Sriracha sauce and cook for 1 minute.
2. Add zucchini noodles, toss until coated in butter, and then continue cooking for 3 to 4 minutes until tender-crisp.
3. Season the zucchini with salt and black pepper and then serve.

Lime and Garlic Chicken Thighs

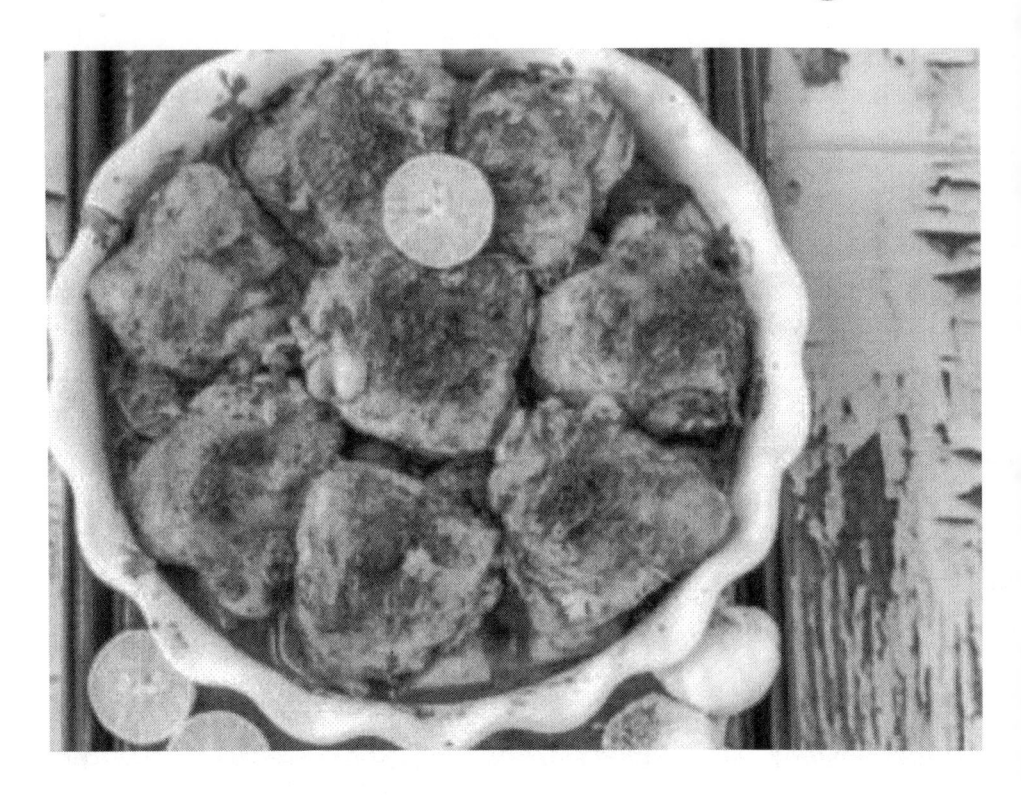

Nutrition Facts Per Serving

Calories	Fats	Proteins	Carbohydrates
572	37.5	54.3	4.3

Ingredients

Serves	1	2	3	4	5	6	7	8
Chicken thigh, large, pasteurized	2	4	6	8	10	12	14	16
Garlic powder, teaspoon	2	4	6	8	10	12	14	16
All-purpose seasoning, teaspoon	2	4	6	8	10	12	14	16
Lime, juiced, zested	1	2	3	4	5	6	7	8
Avocado oil, tablespoon	2	4	6	8	10	12	14	16
Salt, by taste								
Black pepper, by taste								

Instructions

1. Place the chicken thighs in a shallow dish, drizzle with lime juice, and then add garlic powder, lime zest, and all-purpose seasoning.
2. Toss until coated and then let the chicken marinate in the refrigerator for 30 minutes.
3. Then place the oil in a medium skillet pan over medium heat, and when hot, arrange chicken thighs in it and cook for 8 to 10 minutes until thoroughly cooked and tender.
4. Serve directly.

Tuna Salad

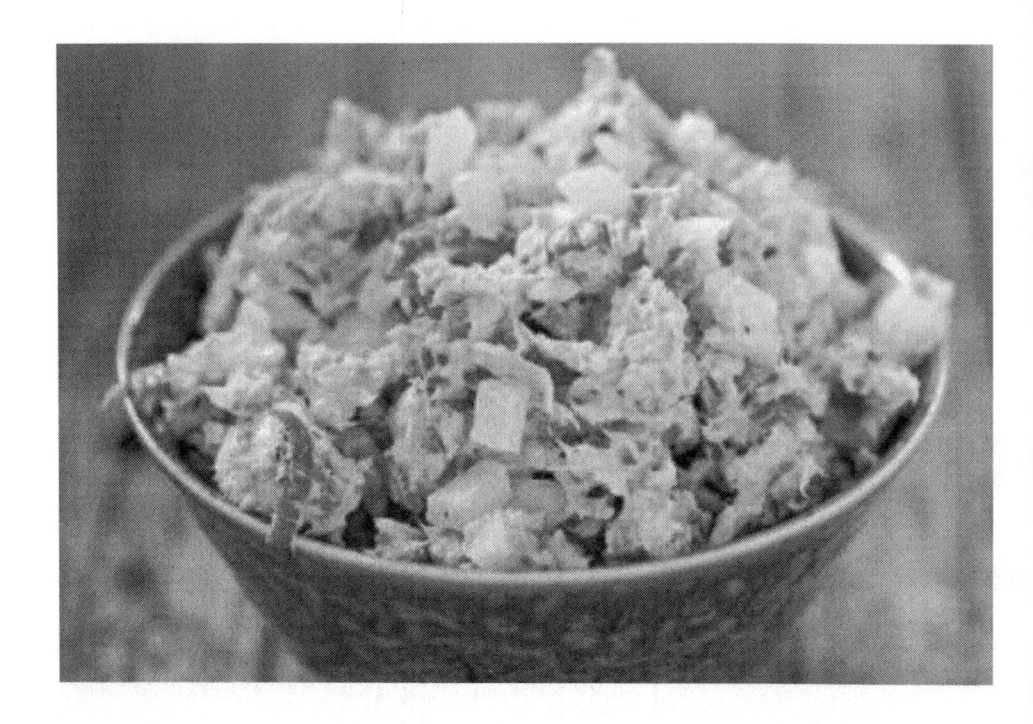

Nutrition Facts Per Serving

Calories	Fats	Proteins	Carbohydrates
548	39.6	46.6	1.4

Ingredients

Serves	1	2	3	4	5	6	7	8
Tuna, canned, drained, ounces	12	24	36	48	60	72	84	96
Chili and garlic sauce, tablespoon	2	4	6	8	10	12	14	16
Sesame seeds, teaspoon	1	2	3	4	5	6	7	8
Mayonnaise, tablespoon	2	4	6	8	10	12	14	16
Sesame oil, tablespoon	1	2	3	4	5	6	7	8
Red pepper flakes, teaspoon	¼	½	¾	1	1¼	1½	1¾	2

Instructions

1. Place the chili and garlic sauce in a medium bowl, add mayonnaise, oil and red pepper flakes, and then whisk until combined.
2. Add tuna, toss until combined, sprinkle with sesame seeds, and then let the salad chill in the refrigerator for 30 minutes.
3. Serve ASAP.

Cheesy Deviled Eggs with Avocado

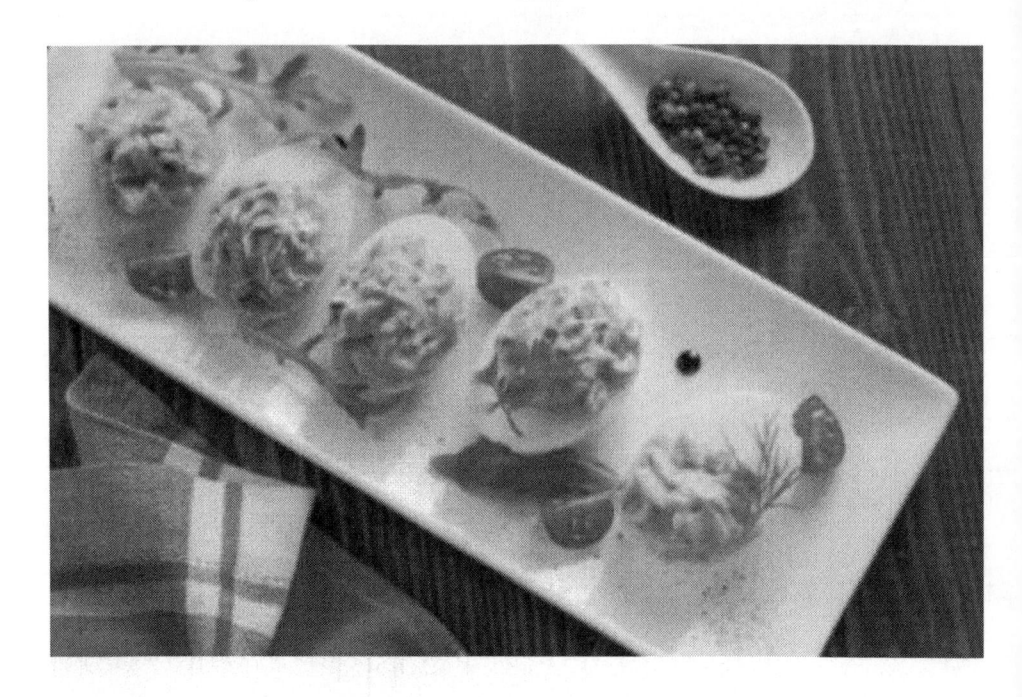

Nutrition Facts Per Serving

Calories	Fats	Proteins	Carbohydrates
337	28.5	16	4.2

Ingredients

Serves	1	2	3	4	5	6	7	8
Eggs, pasteurized, boiled	2	4	6	8	10	12	14	16
Avocado, peeled, pitted, mashed	¼	½	¾	1	1¼	1½	1¾	2
Mozzarella cheese, grated, full-fat, teaspoon	1	2	3	4	5	6	7	8
Mustard paste, teaspoon	½	1	1½	2	2½	3	3½	4
Mayonnaise, tablespoon	1	2	3	4	5	6	7	8
Salt, by taste								
Black pepper, by taste								

Instructions

1. Peel the eggs, cut each in half lengthwise, and then spoon the egg yolk into a small bowl.
2. Add the remaining ingredients into the egg yolks and then stir until well mixed.
3. Spoon the egg yolk mixture evenly into the eggs and then serve.

Ranch Deviled Eggs

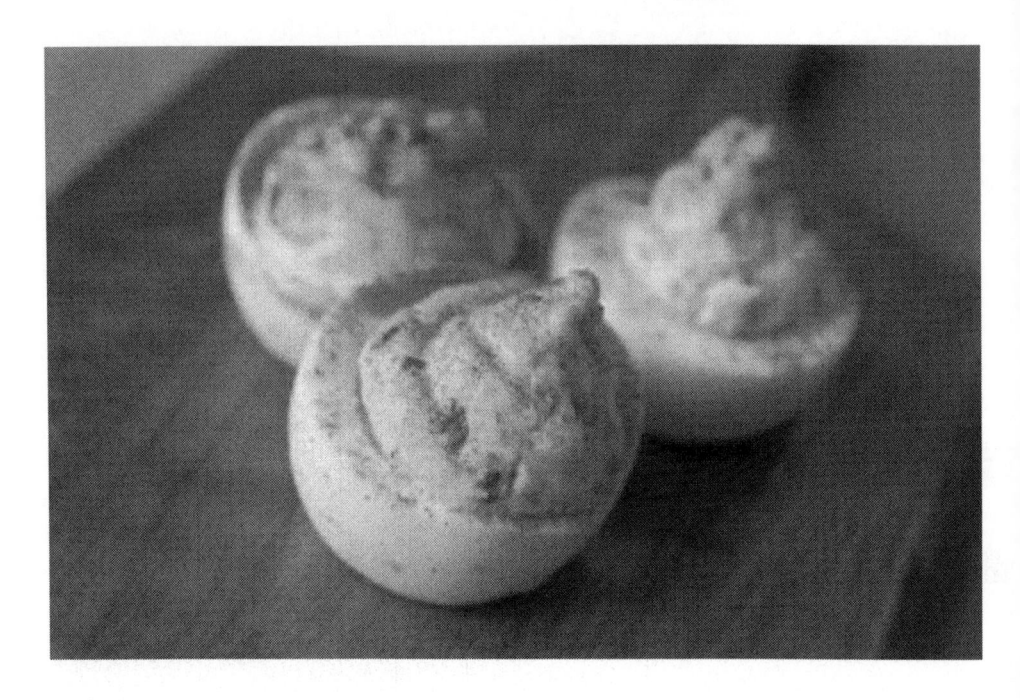

Nutrition Facts Per Serving

Calories	Fats	Proteins	Carbohydrates
437	39.8	17.5	2.2

Ingredients

Serves	1	2	3	4	5	6	7	8
Eggs, pasteurized, boiled	2	4	6	8	10	12	14	16
Ranch dressing, teaspoon	1	2	3	4	5	6	7	8
Mayonnaise, tablespoon	1 ½	3	4 ½	6	7 ½	9	10 ½	12
Mustard paste, teaspoon	1	2	3	4	5	6	7	8
Bacon slice, pasteurized	1	2	3	4	5	6	7	8
Paprika, by taste								

Instructions

1. Take a medium skillet pan, place it over medium heat, and when hot, add a bacon slice.
2. Cook for 2 to 3 minutes per side until tender-crisp; and when done, let the bacon cool for 5 minutes and then chop it.
3. Peel the eggs, cut each in half lengthwise, and then spoon the egg yolk into a small bowl.
4. Add the remaining ingredients into the egg yolks and then stir until well mixed.
5. Spoon the egg yolk mixture evenly into the egg white, top with chopped bacon, and then serve.

Caprese Salad

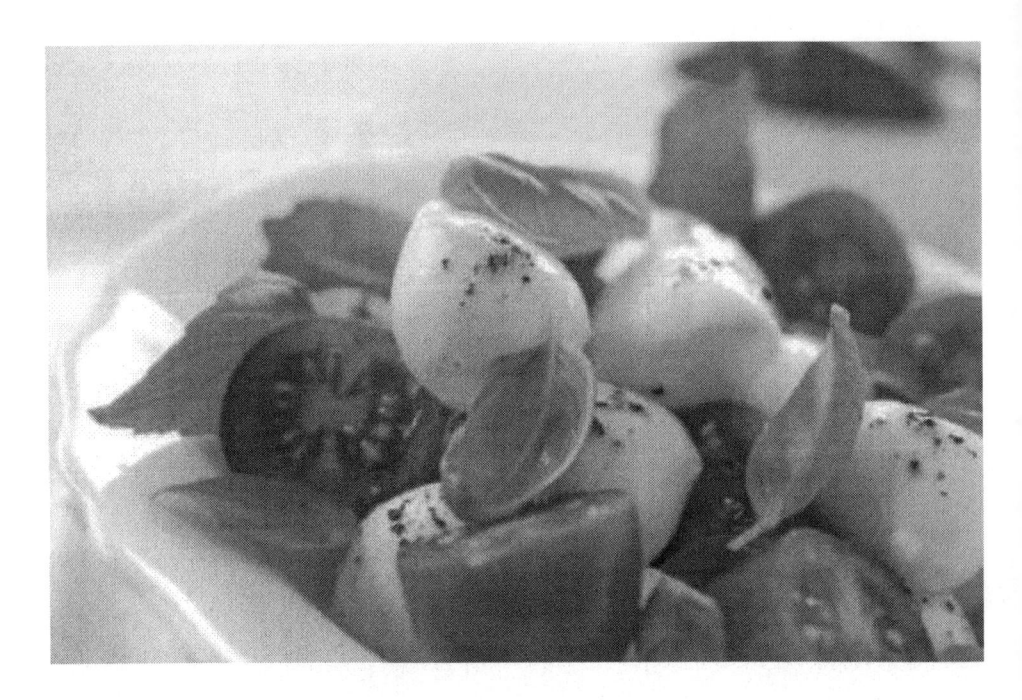

Nutrition Facts Per Serving

Calories	Fats	Proteins	Carbohydrates
464	37.1	26.7	5.8

Ingredients

Serves	1	2	3	4	5	6	7	8
Cherry tomatoes, ounces	4	8	12	16	20	24	28	32
Basil leaves, fresh, chopped, cup	¼	½	¾	1	1¼	1½	1¾	2
Mozzarella cheese, block, ounces	4	8	12	16	20	24	28	32
Avocado oil, teaspoon	2	4	6	8	10	12	14	16
Salt, by taste								
Black pepper, by taste								

Instructions

1. Cut each cherry tomato in half and add to a salad bowl.
2. Chop the mozzarella cheese into bite-size pieces and add to the salad bowl along with basil leaves.
3. Drizzle with oil, sprinkle with salt and black pepper, and then toss until combined.
4. Serve punctually.

Marinara Deviled Egg

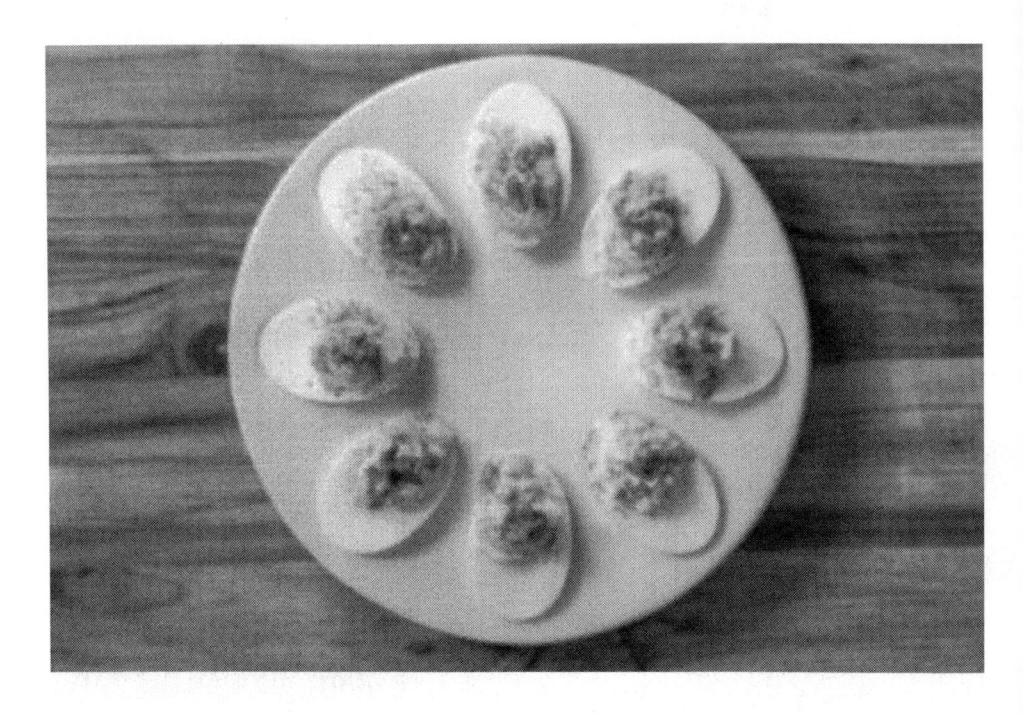

Nutrition Facts Per Serving

Calories	Fats	Proteins	Carbohydrates
266	22.2	14	2.7

Ingredients

Serves	1	2	3	4	5	6	7	8
Eggs, pasteurized, boiled	2	4	6	8	10	12	14	16
Lime juice, teaspoon	1	2	3	4	5	6	7	8
Chipotle hot sauce, tablespoon	1	2	3	4	5	6	7	8
Marinara sauce, tablespoon	1	2	3	4	5	6	7	8
Mayonnaise, tablespoon	1	2	3	4	5	6	7	8
Black pepper, by taste								

Instructions

1. Peel the eggs, cut each in half lengthwise, and then spoon the egg yolk into a small bowl.
2. Add the remaining ingredients into the egg yolks and then stir until well mixed.
3. Spoon the egg yolk mixture evenly into the egg whites and then serve.

Asparagus and Tomato Salad

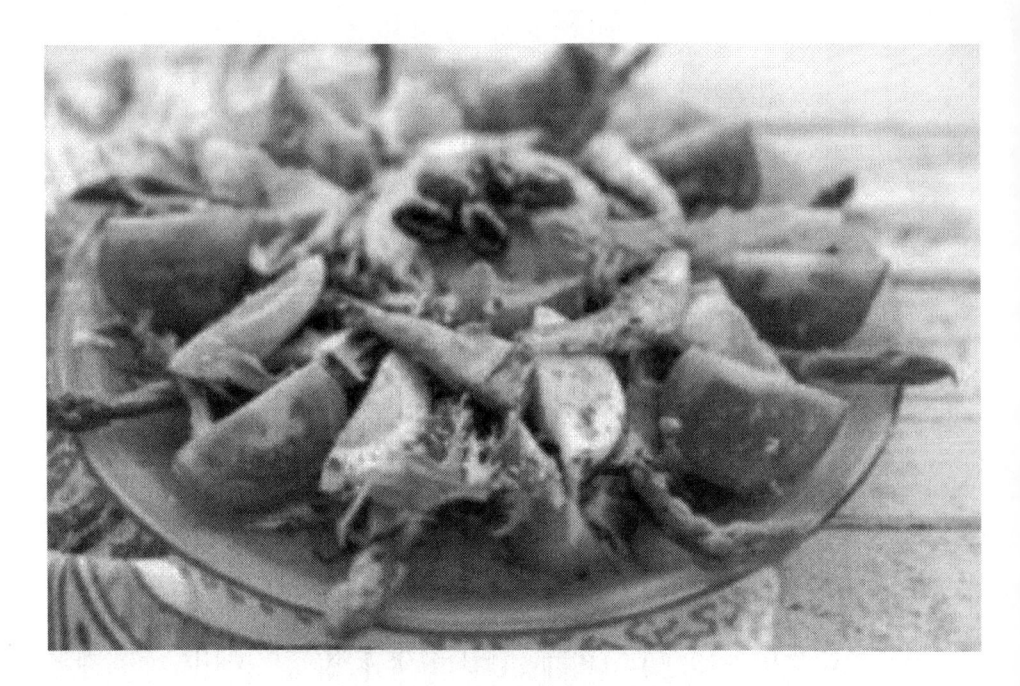

Nutrition Facts Per Serving

Calories	Fats	Proteins	Carbohydrates
516	47	18.1	5.2

Ingredients

Serves	1	2	3	4	5	6	7	8
Asparagus, canned, drain, ounces	2	4	6	8	10	12	14	16
Cherry tomato, ounces	3	6	9	12	15	18	21	24
Pecans, tablespoons	2	4	6	8	10	12	14	16
Egg, pasteurized, boiled	1	2	3	4	5	6	7	8
Avocado oil, tablespoon	2	4	6	8	10	12	14	16
Apple cider vinegar, tablespoon	1	2	3	4	5	6	7	8
Salt, by taste								

Instructions

1. Cut each cherry tomato in half, place it in a salad bowl, and then add the asparagus and pecans.
2. Peel the boiled eggs, cut it into slices, and add them to the salad bowl.
3. Pour the oil into a small bowl, add vinegar, and then stir until combined.
4. Pour the vinegar-oil mixture over salad, season with salt, and then toss gently until mixed.
5. Serve promptly.

Pork and Egg Cup

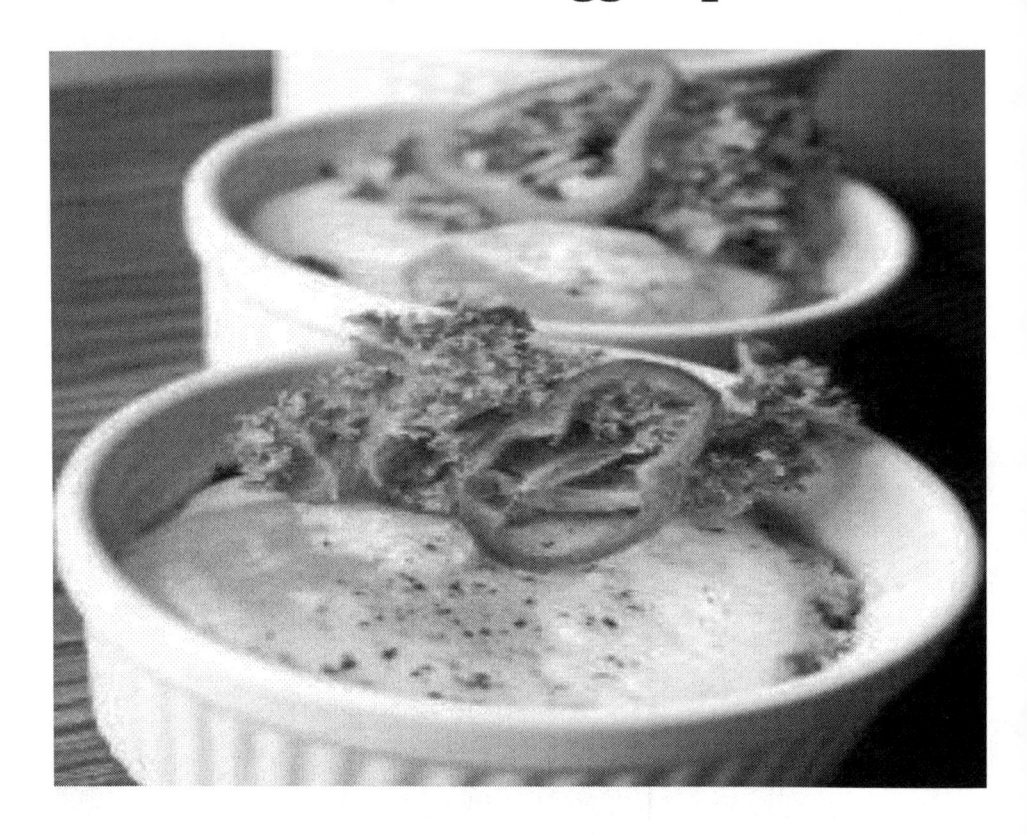

Nutrition Facts Per Serving

Calories	Fats	Proteins	Carbohydrates
354	31.5	16.8	0.9

Ingredients

Serves	1	2	3	4	5	6	7	8
Pork sausage, ounces	2	4	6	8	10	12	14	16
Egg, pasteurized	1	2	3	4	5	6	7	8
Cheddar cheese, grated	1	2	3	4	5	6	7	8
Salt, by taste								
Black pepper, by taste								

Instructions

1. Switch on the oven, then set it to 350 degrees F, and let it preheat.
2. In the meantime, place a skillet pan over medium heat, add sausage, crumble it, and then cook for 3 to 4 minutes or until beginning to brown.
3. Drain any excess fat, add salt, black pepper, and cheese, stir until mixed, and then spoon the mixture into a ramekin.
4. Carefully crack the egg over the sausage mixture, season with some more salt and black pepper, and then bake for 10 minutes or more until the egg has cooked.
5. Serve ASAP.

Berries in Yogurt Cream

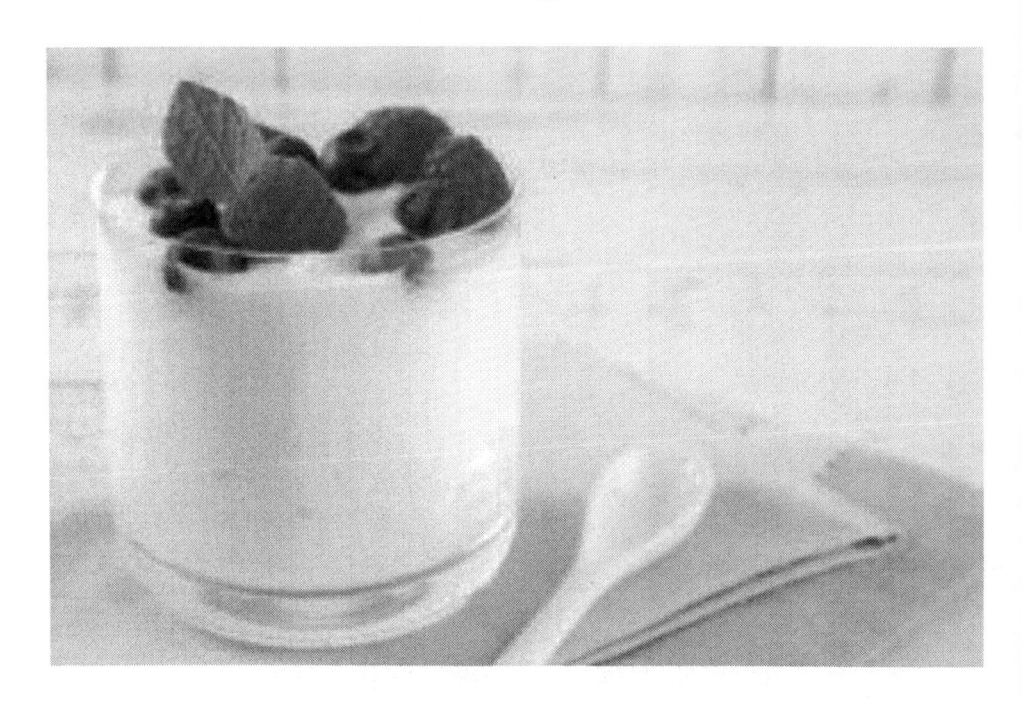

Nutrition Facts Per Serving

Calories	Fats	Proteins	Carbohydrates
468	42.6	15.2	5.9

Ingredients

Serves	1	2	3	4	5	6	7	8
Blackberries, fresh, ounces	½	1	1½	2	2½	3	3½	4
Raspberries, fresh, ounces	½	1	1½	2	2½	3	3½	4
Yogurt, full-fat, ounces	2	4	6	8	10	12	14	16
Heavy cream, full-fat, ounces	2	4	6	8	10	12	14	16
Erythritol sweetener, tablespoon	1	2	3	4	5	6	7	8

Instructions

1. Place the yogurt in a medium bowl, add cream, and then whisk until combined.
2. Sprinkle erythritol over the yogurt mixture, don't stir, then cover the top with a lid, and let it rest in the refrigerator for 1 hour or more until chilled.
3. Then add the berries and serve.

DINNER

Shrimp and Bacon

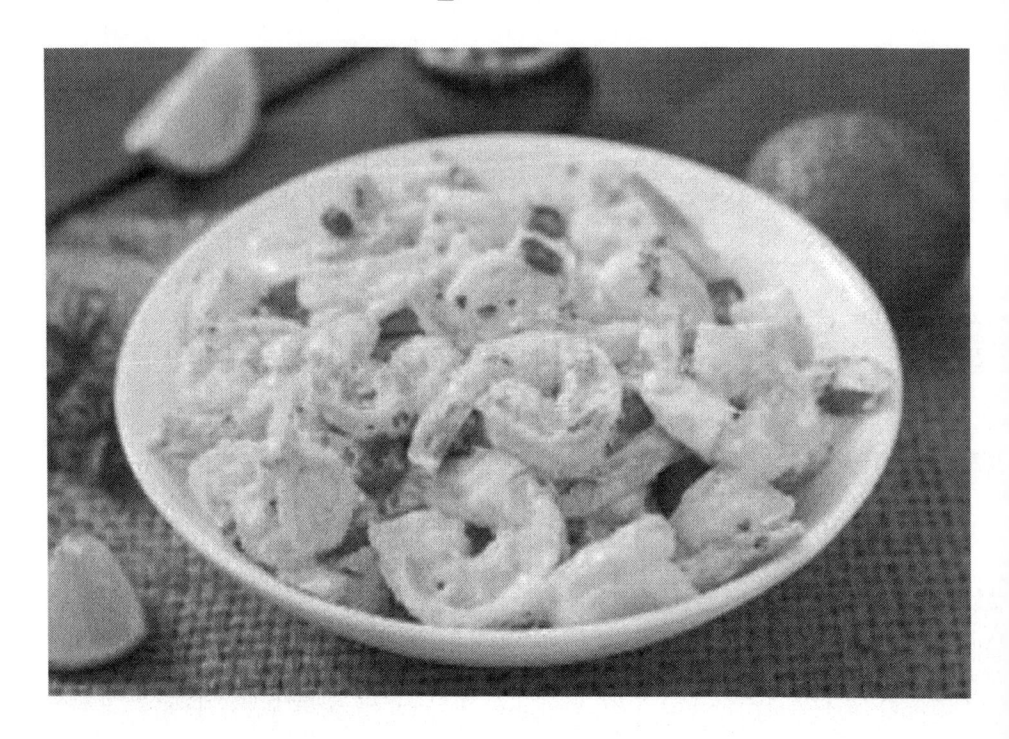

Nutrition Facts Per Serving

Calories	Fats	Proteins	Carbohydrates
297	24.4	17.8	1.5

Ingredients

Serves	1	2	3	4	5	6	7	8
Bacon slice, pasteurized, chopped	2	4	6	8	10	12	14	16
Shrimps, peeled, deveined, ounces	4	8	12	16	20	24	28	32
Heavy cream, full-fat, ounces	3	6	9	12	15	18	21	24
Avocado oil, tablespoon	1	2	3	4	5	6	7	8
Salt, by taste								
Black pepper, by taste								

Instructions

1. Place a medium skillet pan over medium heat and when hot, add the chopped bacon and cook for 4 to 5 minutes per side until tender-crisp.
2. Add the oil into the pan, and when hot, add the shrimps.
3. Season them with black pepper and salt, and then continue cooking for 5 minutes or more until shrimps turn pink.
4. Add the cream into the pan, stir until coated, switch the heat to the low level, and then continue cooking for 1 minute or until hot.
5. Serve punctually.

Chili

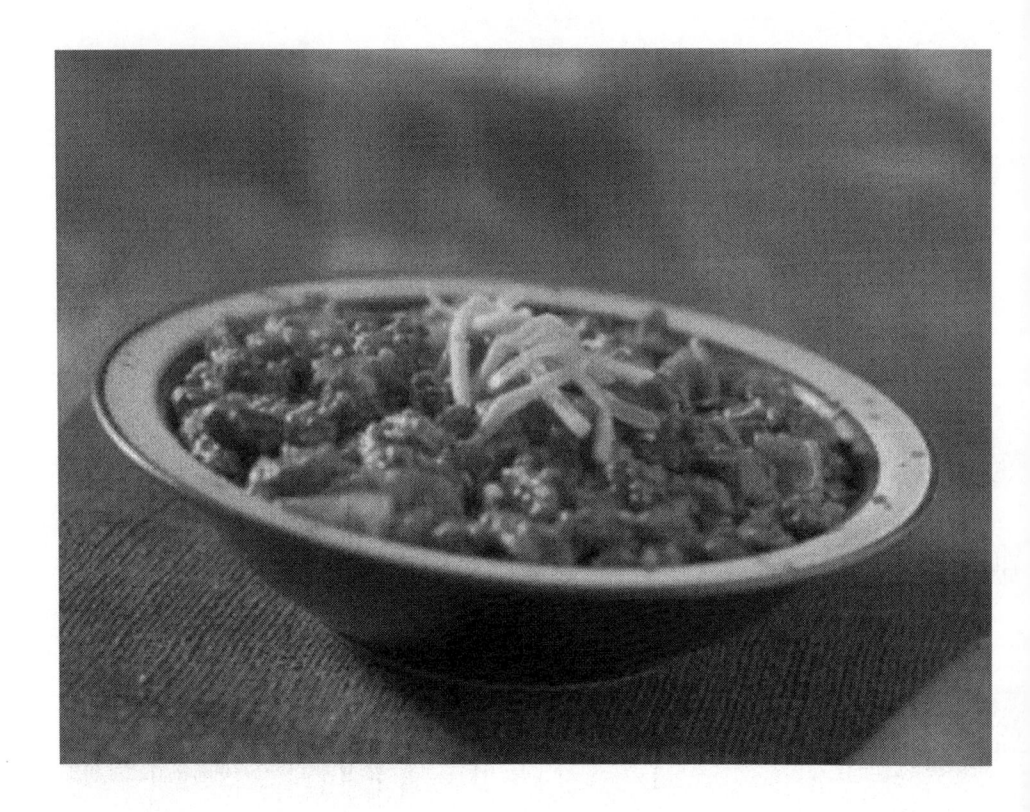

Nutrition Facts Per Serving

Calories	Fats	Proteins	Carbohydrates
396	26.4	33.7	5.9

Ingredients

Serves	1	2	3	4	5	6	7	8
Ground beef, ounces	4	8	12	16	20	24	28	32
Jalapeno pepper, chopped	1	2	3	4	5	6	7	8
Tomato sauce, ounces	4	8	12	16	20	24	28	32
Avocado oil, tablespoon	1	2	3	4	5	6	7	8
Water, cup	½	1	1½	2	2½	3	3½	4
Salt, by taste								
Red chili powder, by taste								

Instructions

1. Place the oil in a medium skillet pan over medium heat. Next, when hot, add the beef, crumble it, and then cook for 5 minutes or more until nicely brown.
2. Add the jalapeno pepper, season with salt and red chili powder, stir until mixed, and then continue cooking for 2 minutes until hot.
3. Pour in water and tomato sauce, bring the chili to simmer, and then cook for 15 to 20 minutes until thickened.
4. Taste the chili to adjust seasoning and then serve.

Pumpkin Soup

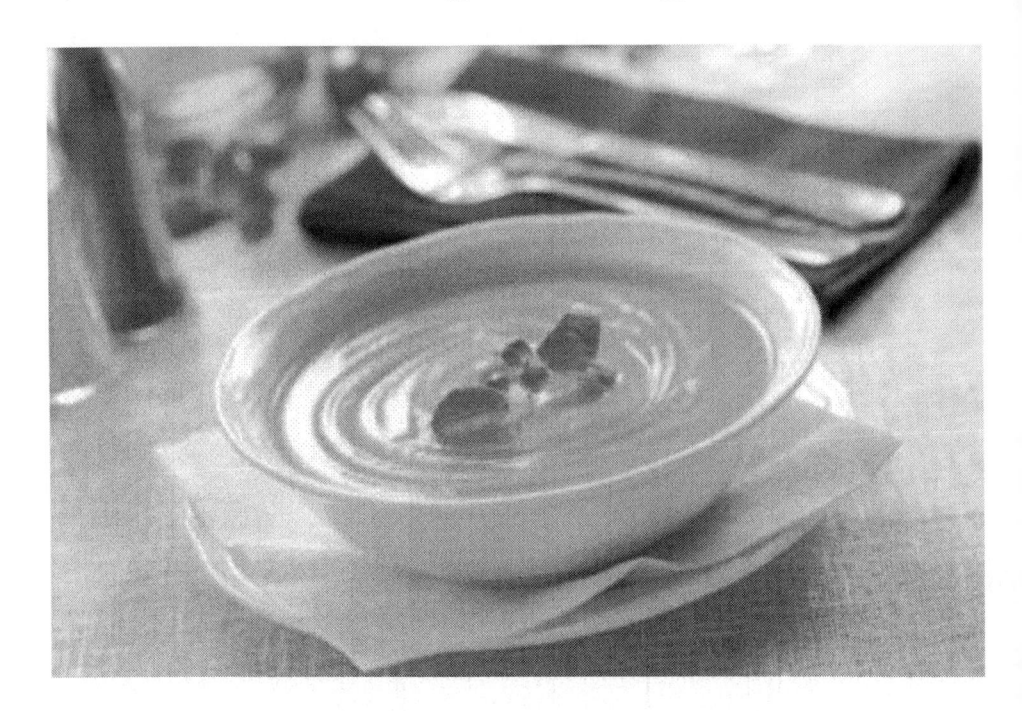

Nutrition Facts Per Serving

Calories	Fats	Proteins	Carbohydrates
605	55.1	19.7	7.6

Ingredients

Serves	1	2	3	4	5	6	7	8
Green beans, canned, drained, ounces	3.5	7	10.5	14	17.5	21	24.5	28
Bacon slices, chopped	2	4	6	8	10	12	14	16
Butter, unsalted, tablespoon	3	6	9	12	15	18	21	24
Cheddar cheese, grated, full-fat, tablespoon	2	4	6	8	10	12	14	16
Garlic powder, teaspoon	½	1	1½	2	2½	3	3½	4
Salt, by taste								
Black pepper, by taste								

Instructions

1. Place a medium skillet pan over medium heat; and when hot, add the chopped bacon and cook for 4 to 5 minutes per side until tender-crisp.
2. Transfer the bacon to a bowl, add butter, and let it melt.
3. Then add the green beans, toss until coated, season with garlic powder, salt, and black pepper. Then cook for 2 minutes until tender-crisp and hot.
4. Spoon the green beans with butter to a heatproof dish, sprinkle bacon and cheese on top, and then broil for 2 minutes until cheese melts.
5. Serve immediately.

Roasted Cauliflower Steaks

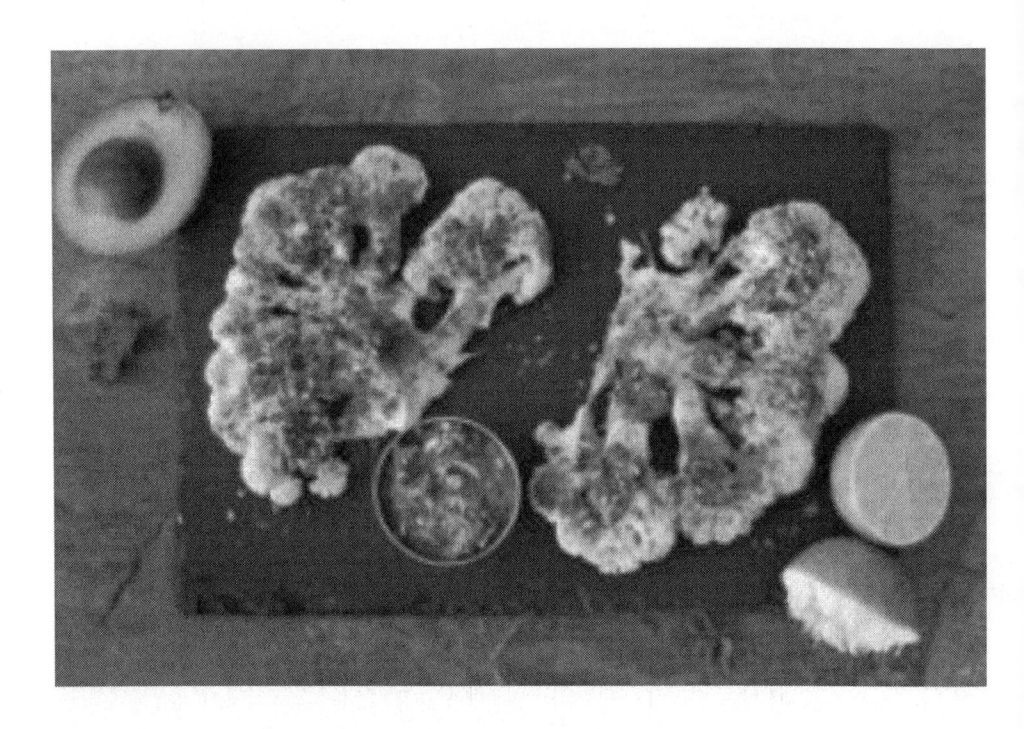

Nutrition Facts Per Serving

Calories	Fats	Proteins	Carbohydrates
383	36.6	9.6	3.8

Ingredients

Serves	1	2	3	4	5	6	7	8
Cauliflower slices, about 2-ounces	2	4	6	8	10	12	14	16
Avocado oil, tablespoon	2	4	6	8	10	12	14	16
Cheddar cheese, grated, tablespoon	4	8	12	16	20	24	28	32
Garlic powder, teaspoon	2	4	6	8	10	12	14	16
Red pepper flakes, to taste								
Salt, by taste								
Black pepper, by taste								

Instructions

1. Switch on the oven, set it to 400 degrees F, and let it preheat.
2. In the meantime, place the oil in a small bowl, add garlic powder, red pepper flakes, salt, and black pepper, and then stir until combined.
3. Brush the oil mixture generously on each side of cauliflower the slices, arrange them on a foil-lined baking sheet, and then bake for 10 minutes.
4. After 10 minutes, flip the cauliflower slices, sprinkle 2 tablespoons cheese on each slice, and then continue baking for 10 minutes until cooked and all cheese melts.
5. Serve immediately.

Bacon Wrapped Chicken

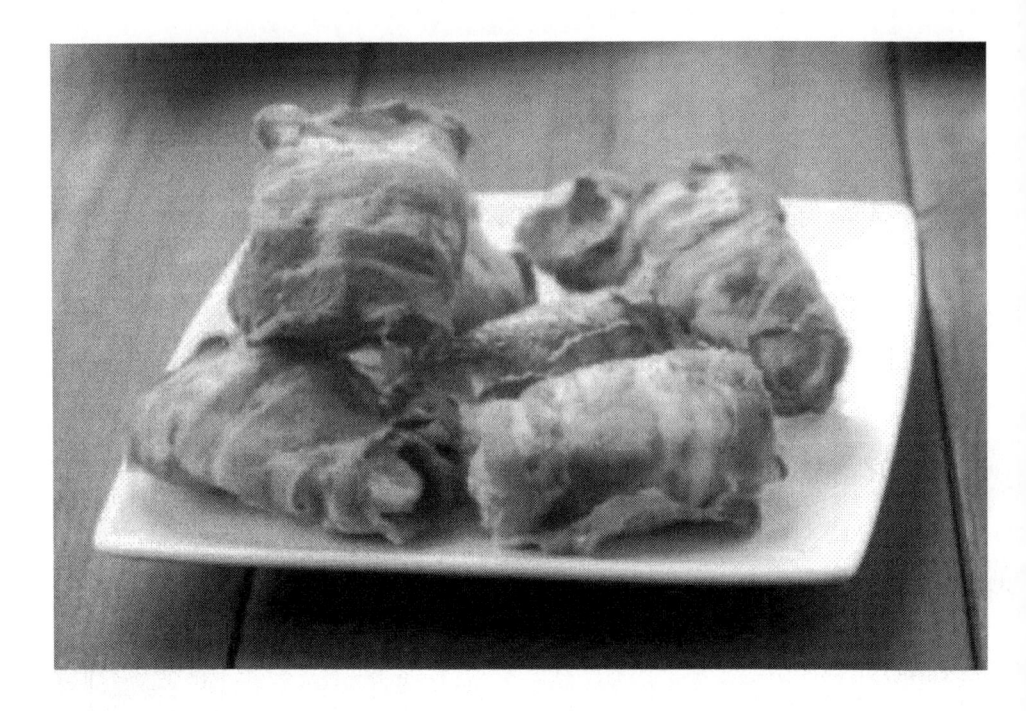

Nutrition Facts Per Serving

Calories	Fats	Proteins	Carbohydrates
580	36.1	62.4	1.5

Ingredients

Serves	1	2	3	4	5	6	7	8
Chicken thighs, pasteurized, large	2	4	6	8	10	12	14	16
Bacon slices, pasteurized	2	4	6	8	10	12	14	16
Cheddar cheese, grated, full-fat	2	4	6	8	10	12	14	16
Garlic powder, by taste								
Paprika, by taste								
Salt, by taste								

Instructions

1. Switch on the oven, then set it to 400 degrees F, and let it preheat.
2. In the meantime, sprinkle garlic, salt, and paprika on both sides of the chicken until coated.
3. Wrap each chicken with a bacon slice, securing with a toothpick, and then arrange each on a greased and foil-lined baking dish.
4. Bake the chicken for 10 minutes per side until cooked; and when done, sprinkle 1 tablespoon cheese over each chicken.
5. Turn on the broiler and continue cooking the chicken for 2 minutes or more until all cheese melts.
6. Serve swiftly.

Teriyaki Chicken

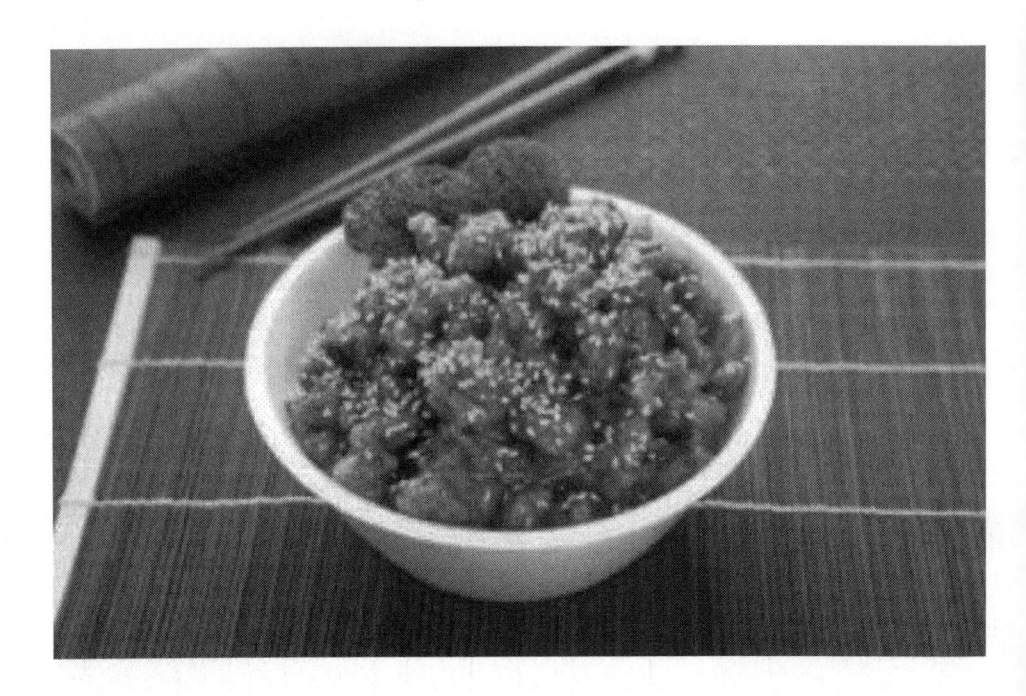

Nutrition Facts Per Serving

Calories	Fats	Proteins	Carbohydrates
580	36.1	62.4	1.5

Ingredients

Serves	1	2	3	4	5	6	7	8
Chicken breast, pasteurized, ounces	4	8	12	16	20	24	28	32
Soy sauce, tablespoon	3	6	9	12	15	18	21	24
Erythritol sweetener, tablespoon	1	2	3	4	5	6	7	8
Avocado oil, tablespoon	1	2	3	4	5	6	7	8
Sesame seeds, teaspoon	1	2	3	4	5	6	7	8

Instructions

1. Place oil in a medium skillet pan over medium heat and let it heat.
2. Cut the chicken into bite-size pieces, add to the skillet pan, and then cook for 5 minutes per side until nicely browned.
3. Sprinkle sweetener over chicken pieces, drizzle with soy sauce, and then stir until mixed.
4. Switch the heat to medium-low level and then continue cooking it for 3 to 4 minutes until the chicken pieces have glazed.
5. Sprinkle sesame seeds over the chicken and then serve.

Coconut Crusted Fish

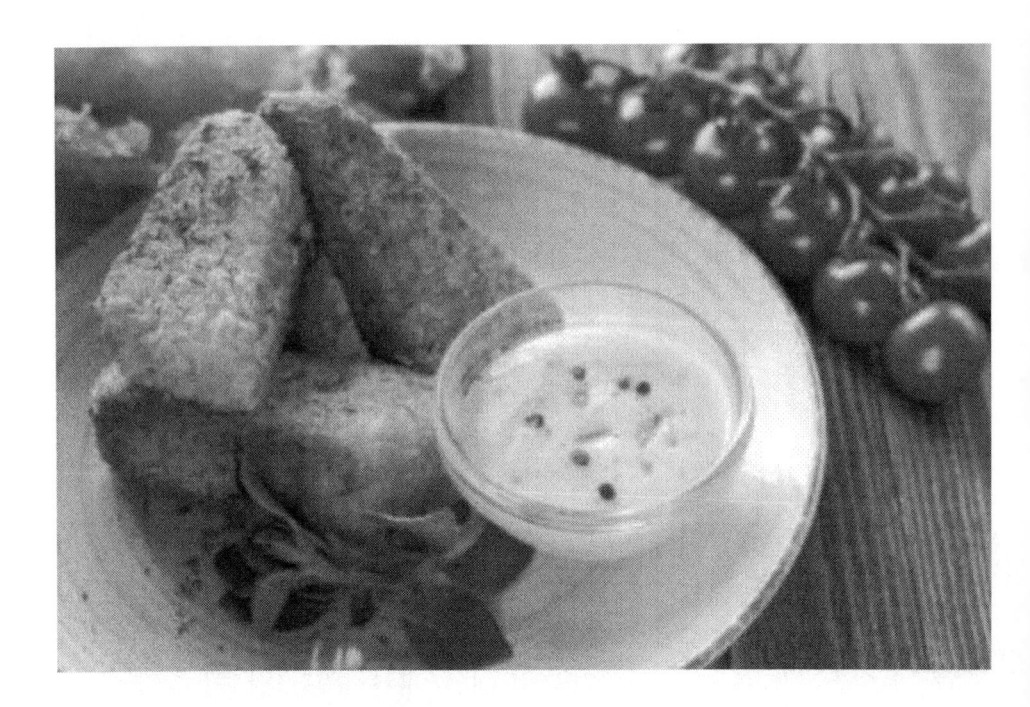

Nutrition Facts Per Serving

Calories	Fats	Proteins	Carbohydrates
958	77.7	55.1	9.6

Ingredients

Serves	1	2	3	4	5	6	7	8
Fillet of white fish, wild-caught, skinless	2	4	6	8	10	12	14	16
Egg, pasteurized	1	2	3	4	5	6	7	8
Coconut flakes, unsweetened, ounces	2	4	6	8	10	12	14	16
Avocado oil, tablespoon	3	6	9	12	15	18	21	24
Salt, by taste								
Black pepper, by taste								

Instructions

1. Place the coconut flakes in a shallow dish, add salt and black pepper, and stir until mixed.
2. Crack the egg in another shallow dish and whisk until frothy.
3. Dip a fish fillet into the egg, dredge and press the fillet into coconut flakes until evenly coated, place on a plate, and then repeat with another fish fillet.
4. Place the oil in a large skillet pan over medium heat and when hot, arrange the fish fillets in it and then cook for 7 to 10 minutes per side until golden brown and cooked.
5. Serve directly.

Red Curry Glazed Fish

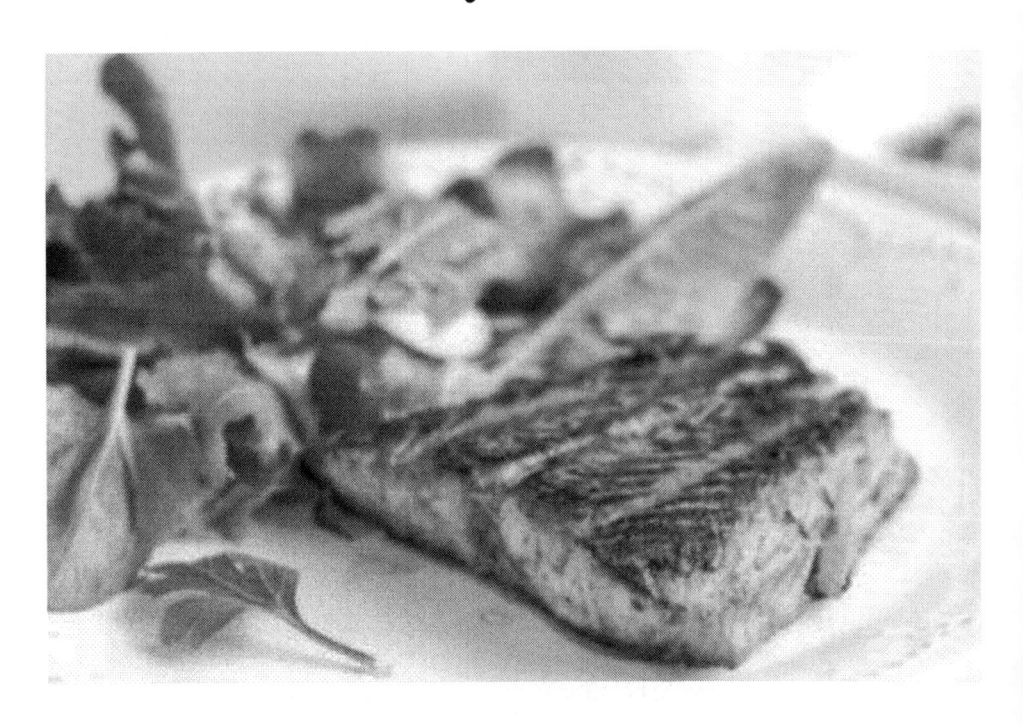

Nutrition Facts Per Serving

Calories	Fats	Proteins	Carbohydrates
283	16.4	30.4	3.5

Ingredients

Serves	1	2	3	4	5	6	7	8
Fillet of white fish, wild-caught, skinless	2	4	6	8	10	12	14	16
Red curry paste, tablespoon	1	2	3	4	5	6	7	8
Avocado oil, tablespoon	1	2	3	4	5	6	7	8
Erythritol sweetener, teaspoon	½	1	1½	2	2½	3	3½	4
Salt, by taste								
Black pepper, by taste								

Instructions

1. Place the oil and red curry paste in a small bowl, add sweetener, salt, and black pepper and stir until mixed.
2. Brush the curry mixture evenly on each side of the fish fillet and then arrange them on a foil-lined baking sheet.
3. Broil the fish for 5 minutes per side until thoroughly cooked and glazed, and then serve.

Beef and Broccoli

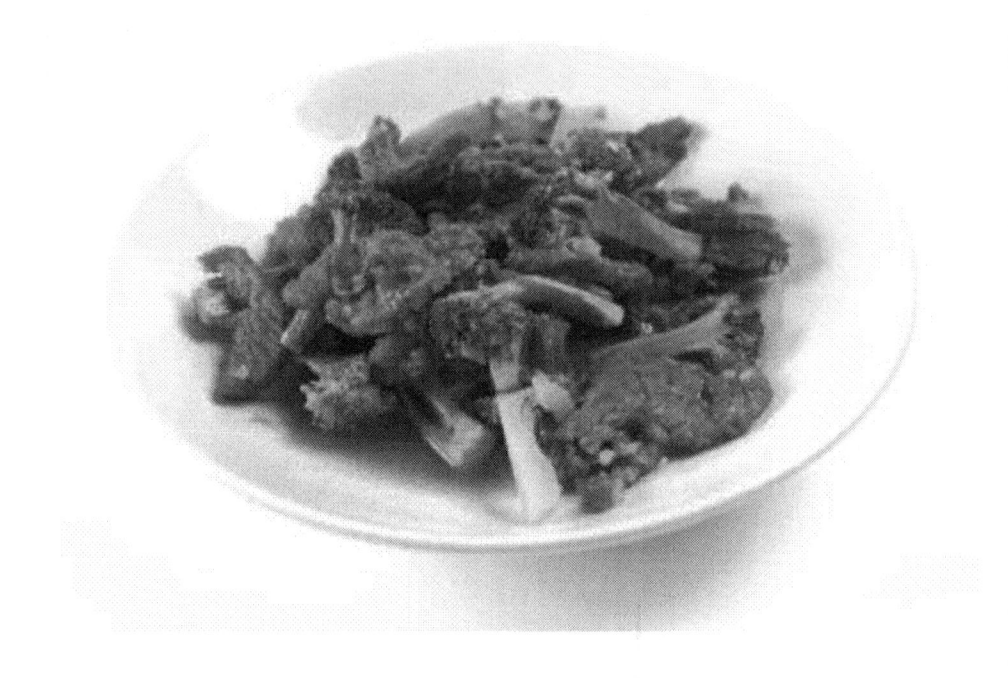

Nutrition Facts Per Serving

Calories	Fats	Proteins	Carbohydrates
370	30	20.4	4.6

Ingredients

Serves	1	2	3	4	5	6	7	8
Beef steak, grass-fed, ounces	2	4	6	8	10	12	14	16
Broccoli florets, ounces	3	6	9	12	15	18	21	24
Avocado oil, tablespoon	2	4	6	8	10	12	14	16
Chicken broth, tablespoon	4	8	12	16	20	24	28	32
Soy sauce, tablespoon	2	4	6	8	10	12	14	16
Salt, by taste								
Black pepper, by taste								

Instructions

1. Place 1 tablespoon oil in a medium skillet pan over medium heat, and let it heat.
2. Cut the steak into bite-size pieces, add them to the pan, and then cook for 3 to 4 minutes per side until no longer pink.
3. Transfer the beef pieces to a plate, add the remaining oil and when hot, add remaining ingredients and stir until mixed.
4. Switch the heat to the low level and continue cooking for 4 to 6 minutes until broccoli is almost tender.
5. Add the beef pieces into the pan, toss until mixed, and then cook for 1 minute until hot.
6. Serve right away.

Cheesy Kale Patties

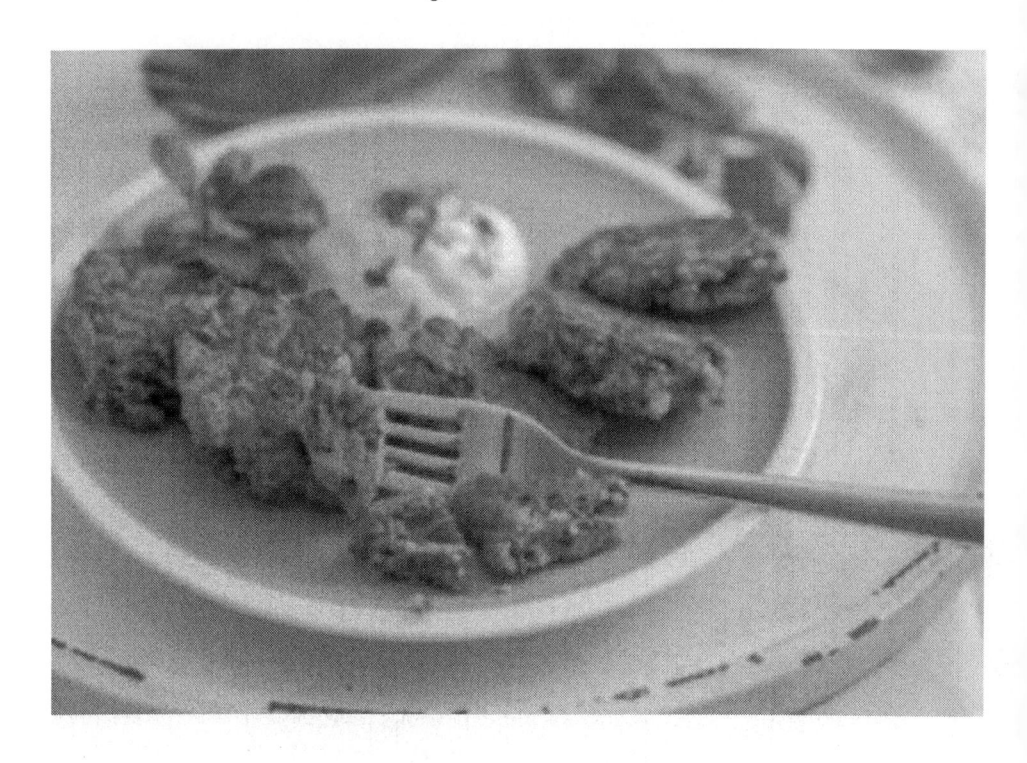

Nutrition Facts Per Serving

Calories	Fats	Proteins	Carbohydrates
498	35.4	42.3	2.5

Ingredients

Serves	1	2	3	4	5	6	7	8
Ground chicken, pasteurized, ounces	6	12	18	24	30	36	42	48
Kale, chopped, cup	½	1	1½	2	2½	3	3½	4
Garlic powder, teaspoon	½	1	1½	2	2½	3	3½	4
Avocado oil, tablespoon	1	2	3	4	5	6	7	8
Parmesan cheese, grated, full-fat, tablespoon	2	4	6	8	10	12	14	16
Salt, by taste								
Black pepper, by taste								

Instructions

1. Place ½ teaspoon oil in a skillet pan over medium heat and when hot, add kale, stir in the garlic powder and then cook it for 2 minutes or more until wilted.
2. Spoon the kale into a medium bowl, add chicken and cheese, and then season with salt and black pepper.
3. Stir until well combined and then shape the mixture into two evenly sized patties.
4. Add all remaining oil into the skillet pan and when hot, arrange the patties in it and then cook for 4 to 5 minutes per side until cooked and golden brown.
5. Serve promptly.

Chicken Nuggets

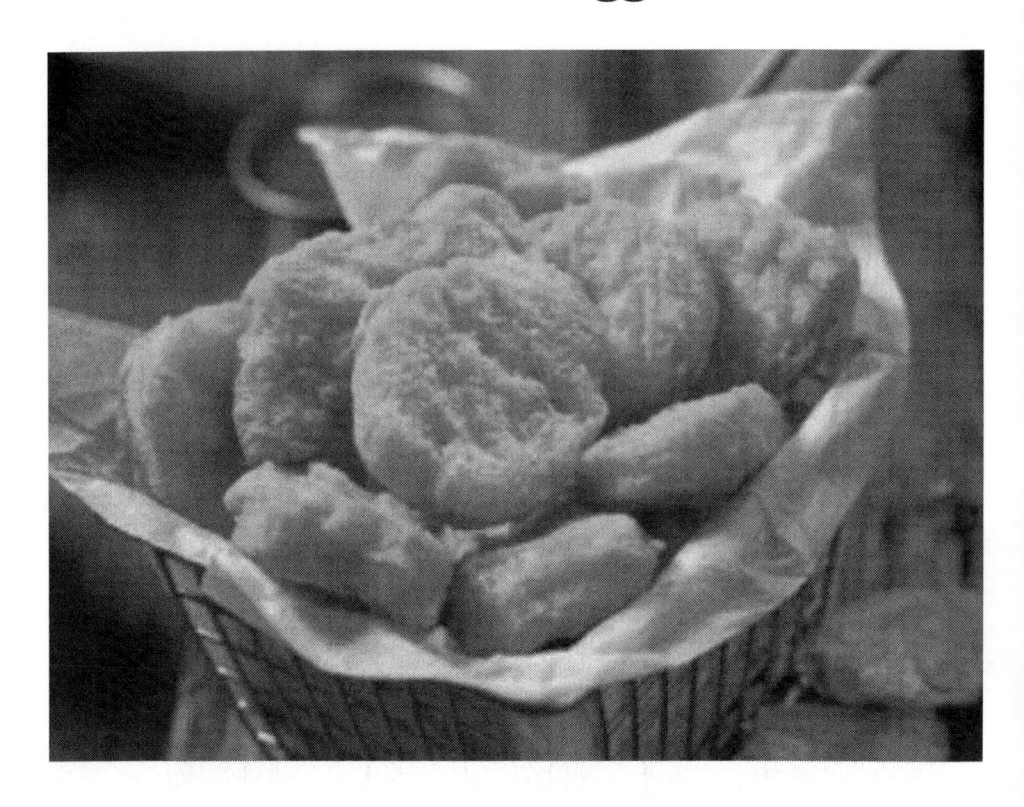

Nutrition Facts Per Serving

Calories	Fats	Proteins	Carbohydrates
870	69.6	52.2	8.7

Ingredients

Serves	1	2	3	4	5	6	7	8
Chicken breast, large, pasteurized	1	2	3	4	5	6	7	8
Almond flour, cup	1/3	2/3	1	1 1/3	1 2/3	2	2 1/3	2 2/3
Mayonnaise, full-fat, tablespoon	3	6	9	12	15	18	21	24
Avocado oil, tablespoon	1	2	3	4	5	6	7	8
Apple cider vinegar, teaspoon	1	2	3	4	5	6	7	8
Salt, by taste								
Black pepper, by taste								

Instructions

1. Pat dry the chicken and then cut into nugget size pieces.
2. Place the flour in a medium bowl, add salt and black pepper, and then stir until mixed.
3. Place the mayonnaise in a medium bowl, add vinegar, and stir until well combined.
4. Working on one chicken piece at a time, coat it into mayonnaise, dredge into the almond flour mixture until evenly coated, and repeat with the other chicken pieces.
5. Place the oil in a medium skillet pan over medium heat, and when hot, arrange all prepared chicken nuggets in it and then cook for 5 minutes per side or more until golden brown and cooked.
6. Serve immediately.

Broccoli and Cheese Soup

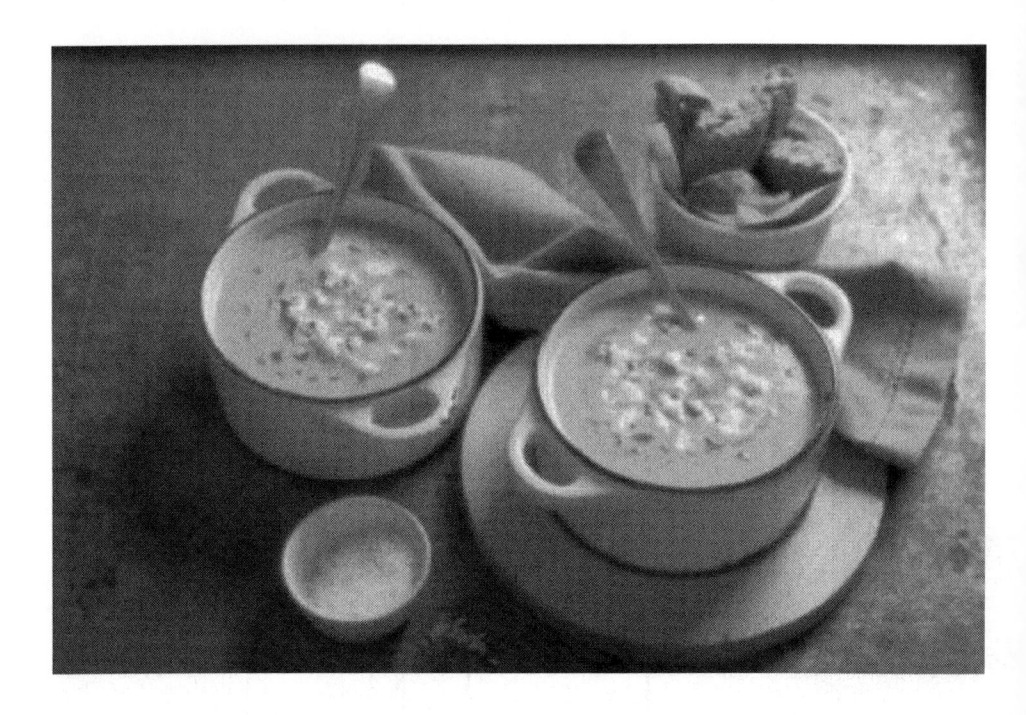

Nutrition Facts Per Serving

Calories	Fats	Proteins	Carbohydrates
595	50.9	26.8	7.4

Ingredients

Serves	1	2	3	4	5	6	7	8
Broccoli florets, cup	1	2	3	4	5	6	7	8
Garlic powder, teaspoon	½	1	1½	2	2½	3	3½	4
Cheddar cheese, grated, full-fat, cup	½	1	1½	2	2½	3	3½	4
Heavy cream, full-fat, cup	1/3	2/3	1	1 1/3	1 2/3	2	2 1/3	2 2/3
Chicken broth, pasteurized, cup	1½	3	4½	6	7½	9	10½	12
Salt, by taste								
Black pepper, by taste								

Instructions

1. Pour the broth in a medium pot, add cream, stir until combined, and then place the pot over medium heat.
2. Add the florets into the pot, season with salt and black pepper, stir until mixed, and then cook for 10 minutes until the florets are tender.
3. Remove the soup from heat, puree it by using an immersion blender until smooth, and then heat it over low heat until hot.
4. Stir in the cheese until it thoroughly melts and then serve.

Cheddar Chicken

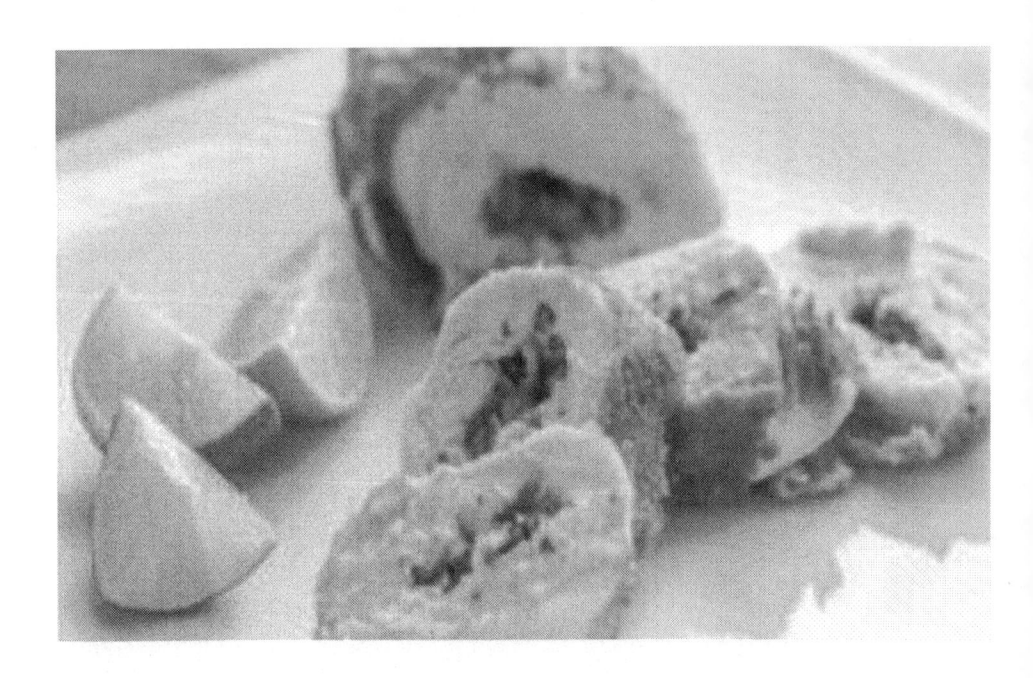

Nutrition Facts Per Serving

Calories	Fats	Proteins	Carbohydrates
383	21.7	46	1

Ingredients

Serves	1	2	3	4	5	6	7	8
Chicken breast, pasteurized, large	1	2	3	4	5	6	7	8
Garlic powder, teaspoon	½	1	1½	2	2½	3	3½	4
Dried basil, teaspoon	½	1	1½	2	2½	3	3½	4
Cheddar cheese, grated, full-fat, tablespoon	1	2	3	4	5	6	7	8
Avocado oil, tablespoon	1	2	3	4	5	6	7	8
Salt, by taste								
Black pepper, by taste								

Instructions

1. Switch on the oven, then set it to 450 degrees F, and let it preheat.
2. Place ½ tablespoon oil in a small bowl, add garlic powder, basil, cheese, salt, and black pepper and stir until combined.
3. Create a pocket in the chicken breast, spoon half of the basil mixture in it, and then brush the remaining mixture generously on all sides of chicken.
4. Place remaining oil into a skillet pan over medium-high heat and when hot, place chicken in it and then cook it for 4 to 5 minutes per side until no longer pink.
5. Transfer the chicken into the pan and then bake it for 10 minutes or more until tender and thoroughly cooked.
6. When done, let the chicken rest for 5 minutes and then serve.

Tuna and Spinach Salad

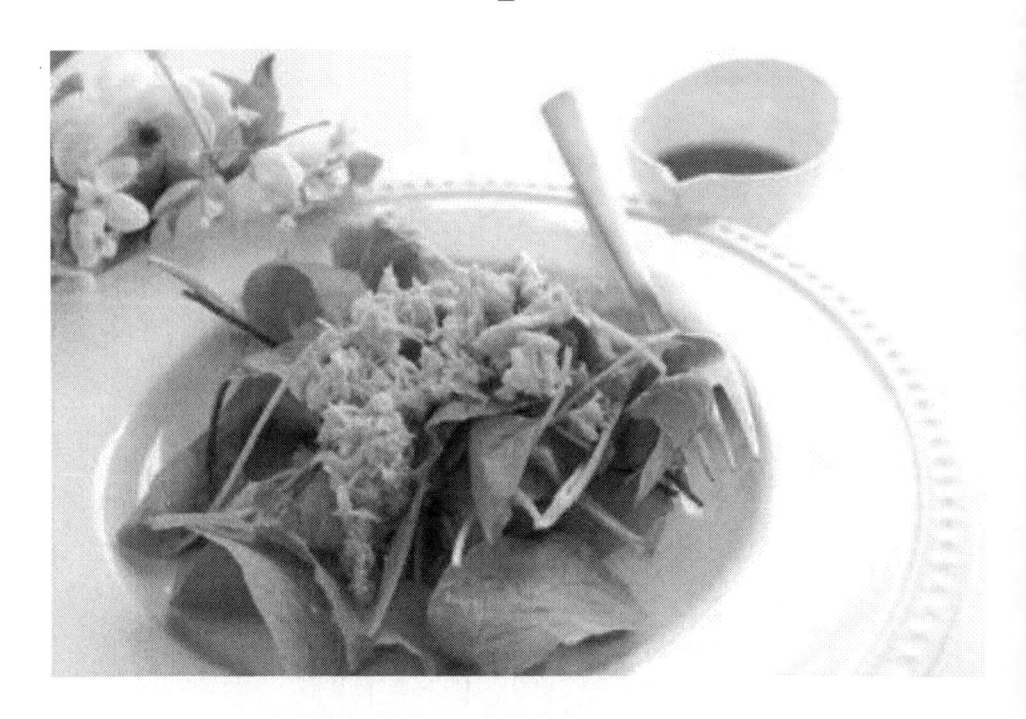

Nutrition Facts Per Serving

Calories	Fats	Proteins	Carbohydrates
703	60.9	35.2	3.5

Ingredients

Serves	1	2	3	4	5	6	7	8
Tuna, canned, drained, ounces	4	8	12	16	20	24	28	32
Spinach, fresh, ounces	2	4	6	8	10	12	14	16
Mozzarella cheese, grated, full-fat, tablespoon	1	2	3	4	5	6	7	8
Mayonnaise, full-fat, cup	1/3	2/3	1	1 1/3	1 2/3	2	2 1/3	2 2/3
Salt, by taste								
Black pepper, by taste								

Instructions

1. Place the mayonnaise in a salad bowl, add salt, black pepper, and cheese, and then stir until smooth.
2. Add the spinach and tuna, toss until coated, and then serve.

Meatloaf

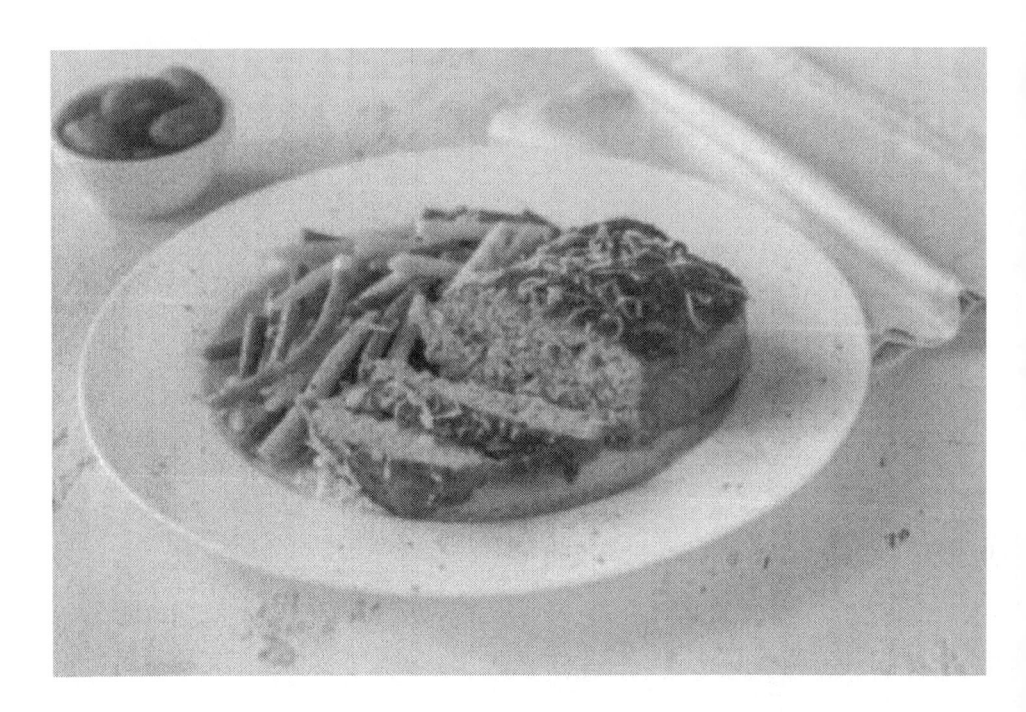

Nutrition Facts Per Serving

Calories	Fats	Proteins	Carbohydrates
504	28	56.7	6.3

Ingredients

Serves	1	2	3	4	5	6	7	8
Ground beef, grass-fed, ounces	6	12	18	24	30	36	42	48
Parmesan cheese, grated, full-fat, tablespoon	2	4	6	8	10	12	14	16
Basil pesto, tablespoon	2	4	6	8	10	12	14	16
Salt, by taste								
Black pepper, by taste								

Instructions

1. Take a large microwave-oven proof mug, place all the ingredients in it, and then stir until well combined.
2. Place the mug into the oven and then microwave for 3 minutes or more at a high heat setting until cooked.
3. Let the meatloaf rest for 1 minute in the mug, then take it out, and serve.

Pulled Chicken

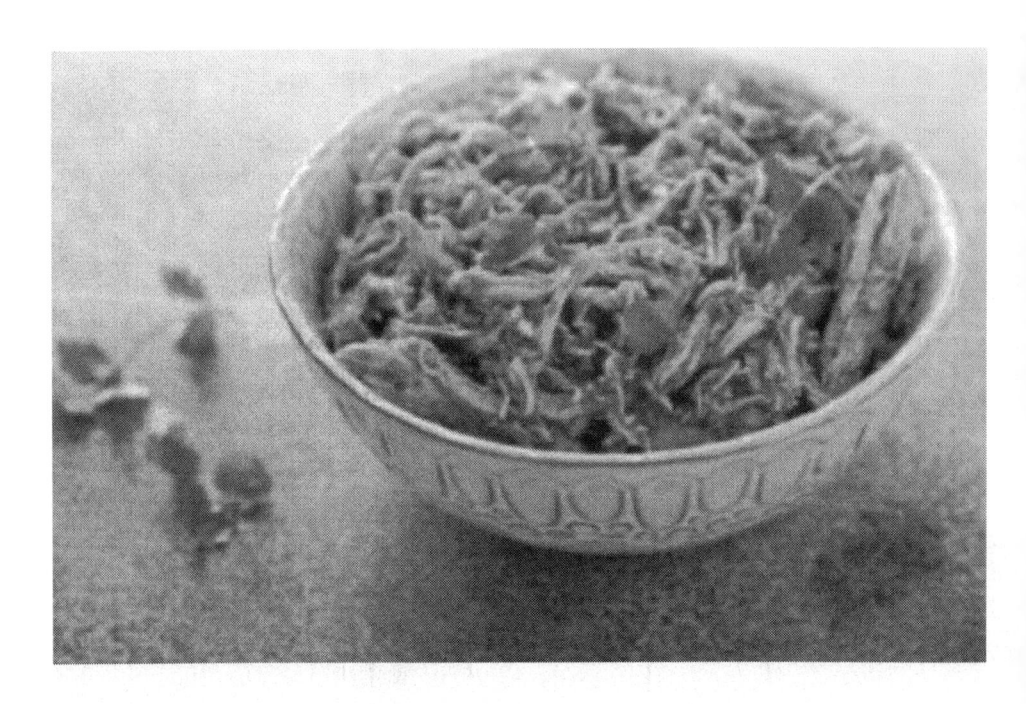

Nutrition Facts Per Serving

Calories	Fats	Proteins	Carbohydrates
708	39.3	86.7	1.8

Ingredients

Serves	1	2	3	4	5	6	7	8
Chicken breast, pasteurized, large	2	4	6	8	10	12	14	16
Garlic powder, teaspoon	½	1	1½	2	2½	3	3½	4
Liquid stevia, tablespoon	1	2	3	4	5	6	7	8
Soy sauce, tablespoon	4	8	12	16	20	24	28	32
Avocado oil, tablespoon	2	4	6	8	10	12	14	16
Water, cup	½	1	1½	2	2½	3	3½	4
Salt, by taste								

Instructions

1. Grease a slow cooker with avocado oil spray and then switch it on.
2. Season the chicken with salt and then place it into the slow cooker.
3. Place the garlic powder in a small bowl, add the remaining ingredients, stir until combined, and then pour this mixture over the chicken.
4. Shut the slow cooker and then cook it for 4 hours at a high heat setting until tender.
5. When done, shred the chicken and then serve.

Buttery Salmon

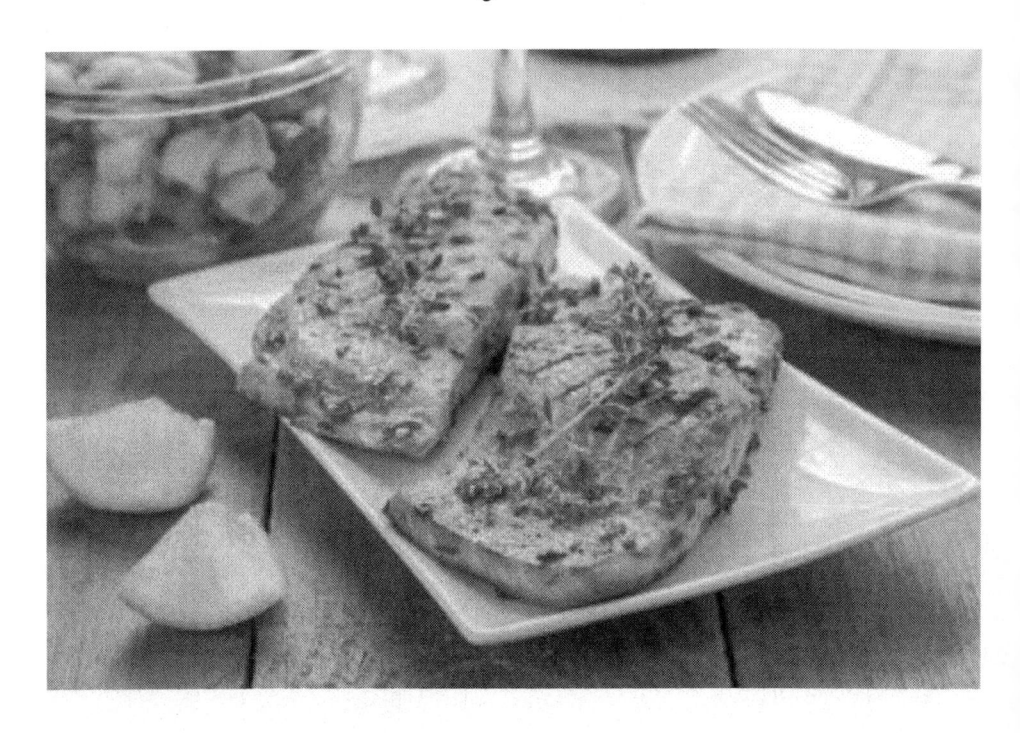

Nutrition Facts Per Serving

Calories	Fats	Proteins	Carbohydrates
506	32.6	51.9	1.3

Ingredients

Serves	1	2	3	4	5	6	7	8
Salmon fillets, skinless	2	4	6	8	10	12	14	16
Garlic powder, teaspoon	1	2	3	4	5	6	7	8
Chopped cilantro, tablespoon	1	2	3	4	5	6	7	8
Butter, unsalted, tablespoon	1	2	3	4	5	6	7	8
Cheddar cheese, grated, full-fat	2	4	6	8	10	12	14	16
Salt, by taste								
Black pepper, by taste								

Instructions

1. Switch on the oven, then set it to 350 degrees F, and let it preheat.
2. Season the salmon with salt and black pepper, and then place the fillets on a rimmed greased baking sheet.
3. Place the cilantro in a small bowl, add butter and cheese, and then stir until combined.
4. Spread the cilantro mixture on the sides of the salmon until coated and then bake for 15 minutes until fork tender.
5. Then turn on the broiler and bake the salmon for 2 to 3 minutes until the top turns a nicely golden brown.
6. Serve immediately.

Salmon with Green Beans

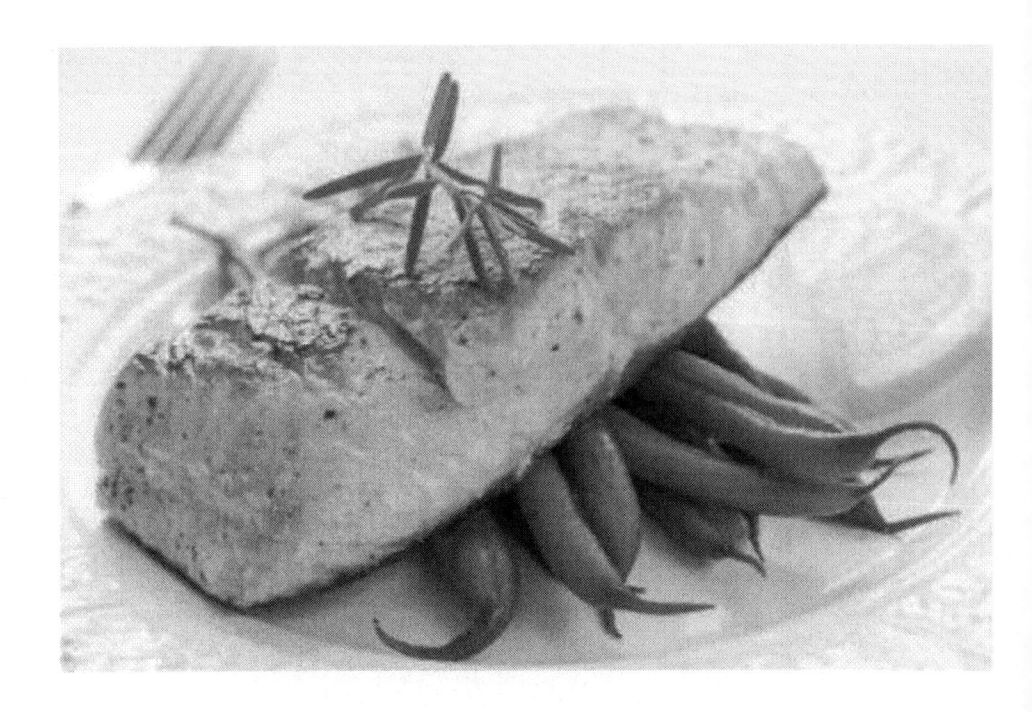

Nutrition Facts Per Serving

Calories	Fats	Proteins	Carbohydrates
622	56.7	24.9	3.1

Ingredients

Serves	1	2	3	4	5	6	7	8
Salmon fillet, skinless	1	2	3	4	5	6	7	8
Green beans, ounces	2	4	6	8	10	12	14	16
Garlic powder, teaspoon	1	2	3	4	5	6	7	8
Butter, unsalted, tablespoon	4	8	12	16	20	24	28	32
Salt, by taste								
Black pepper, by taste								

Instructions

1. Place butter in a frying pan over medium heat, and when it melts, add the salmon fillet to one side of the pan and green beans to the other side of the pan.
2. Season the beans and fish with salt, black pepper, and garlic powder and then cook for 8 to 10 minutes until the salmon has cooked and the beans turn tender-crisp.
3. Serve promptly.

Cream of Asparagus Soup

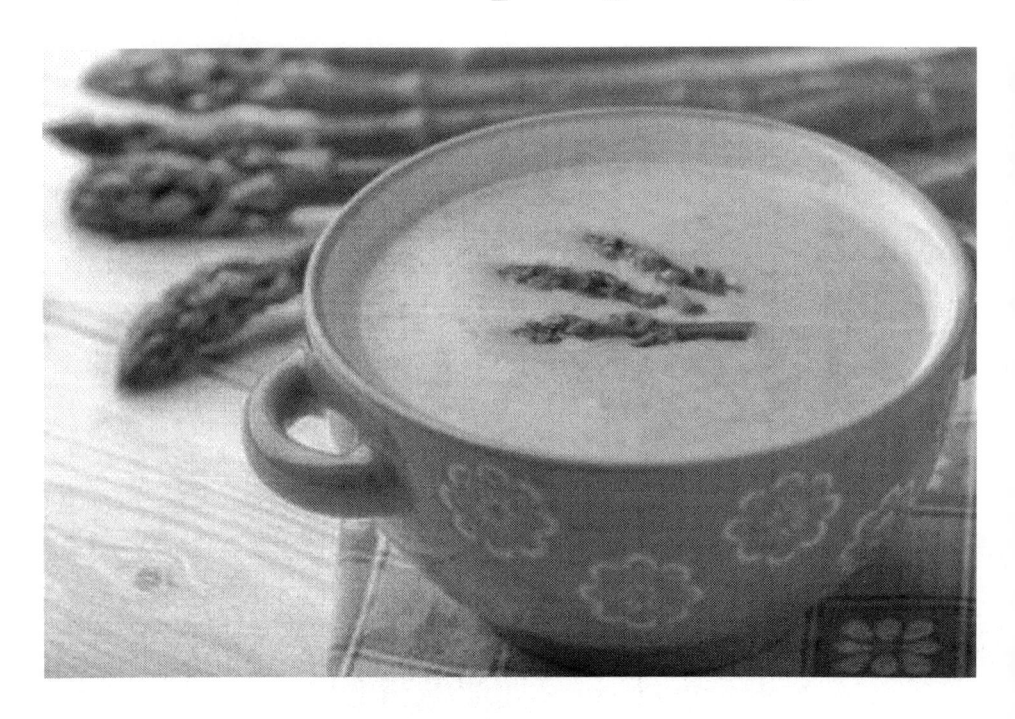

Nutrition Facts Per Serving

Calories	Fats	Proteins	Carbohydrates
467	47.2	4.7	5.8

Ingredients

Serves	1	2	3	4	5	6	7	8
Asparagus, canned, drained, ounces	4	8	12	16	20	24	28	32
Heavy cream, full-fat, ounces	4	8	12	16	20	24	28	32
Garlic powder, teaspoon	1	2	3	4	5	6	7	8
Avocado oil, tablespoon	1	2	3	4	5	6	7	8
Water, cup	1	2	3	4	5	6	7	8
Salt, by taste								
Black pepper, by taste								

Instructions

1. Place the oil in a medium saucepan over medium heat and when hot, add the asparagus.
2. Season with salt and black pepper, cook for 3 to 4 minutes until tender-crisp and bright green.
3. Stir in the garlic powder, cook for 30 seconds or more until fragrant, pour in the water and bring it to boil.
4. Then switch heat to medium-low level, simmer for 10 minutes until the asparagus is tender.
5. Remove the soup from heat, puree it by using an immersion blender until smooth, and then stir in the cream until combined.
6. Serve straight away.

Chicken Salad

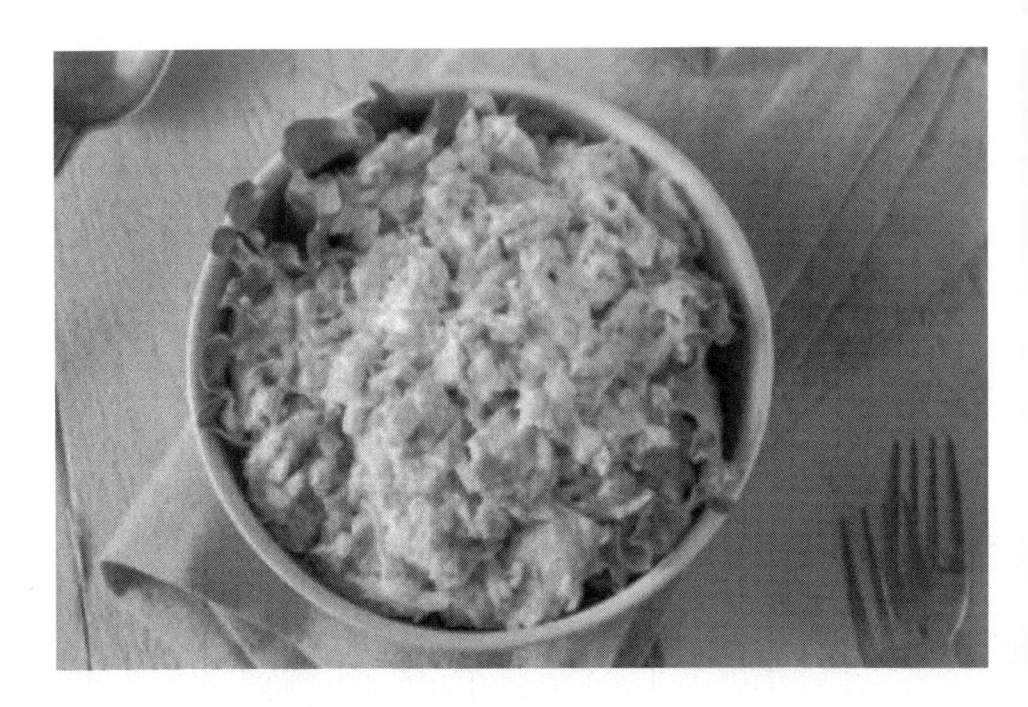

Nutrition Facts Per Serving

Calories	Fats	Proteins	Carbohydrates
394	33	21	3

Ingredients

Serves	1	2	3	4	5	6	7	8
Chicken breast, pasteurized, cooked, shredded	1	2	3	4	5	6	7	8
Egg, pasteurized, boiled	1	2	3	4	5	6	7	8
Dill pickle, chopped, tablespoon	1	2	3	4	5	6	7	8
Mayonnaise, full-fat, cup	¼	½	¾	1	1¼	1½	1¾	2
Apple cider vinegar, teaspoon	1	2	3	4	5	6	7	8
Salt, by taste								
Black pepper, by taste								

Instructions

1. Peel the egg, chop it, and then add it to a salad bowl.
2. Add the pickle, mayonnaise, vinegar, salt, and black pepper and then stir until combined.
3. Fold in the chicken until mixed, chill the salad for 30 minutes in the refrigerator, and then serve.

Bacon-Wrapped Salmon

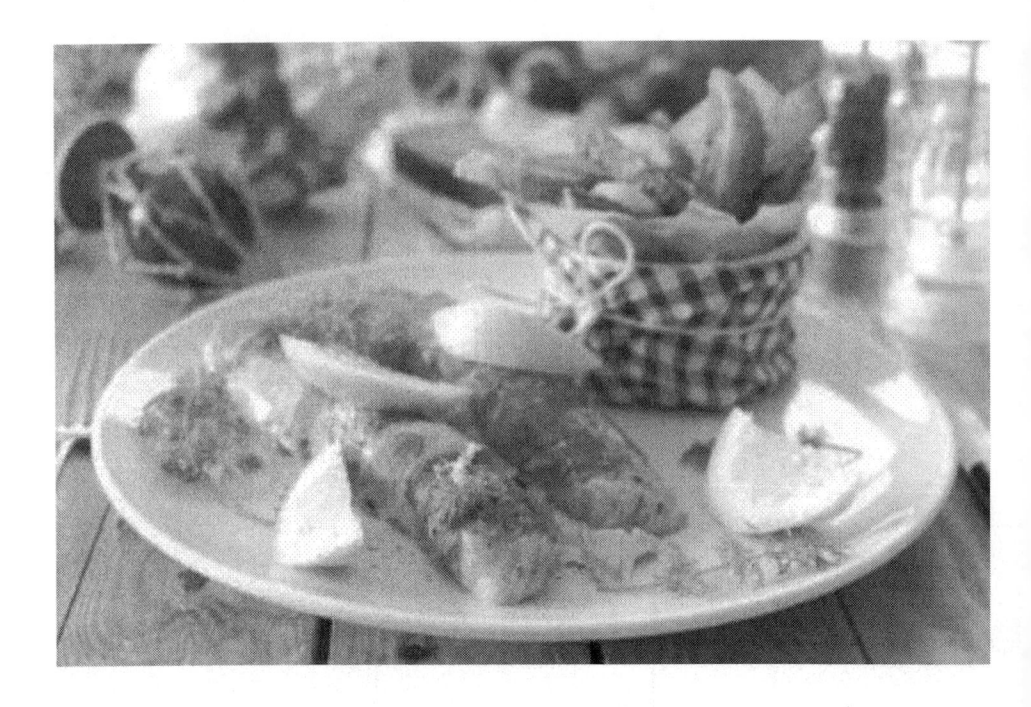

Nutrition Facts Per Serving

Calories	Fats	Proteins	Carbohydrates
730	66.5	31	1.8

Ingredients

Serves	1	2	3	4	5	6	7	8
Salmon fillet, skinless	1	2	3	4	5	6	7	8
Bacon slice, pasteurized	2	4	6	8	10	12	14	16
Avocado oil, tablespoon	1	2	3	4	5	6	7	8
Mayonnaise, full-fat, tablespoon	2	4	6	8	10	12	14	16
Salt, by taste								
Black pepper, by taste								

Instructions

1. Switch on the oven, then set it to 375 degrees F, and let it preheat.
2. In the meantime, place the oil in a skillet pan over medium-high heat and let it heat.
3. Season the salmon with salt and black pepper, wrap with bacon slices, securing with a toothpick, and then cook it for 3 minutes per side until the bacon is tender-crisp.
4. Then bake the salmon in the skillet pan for 5 minutes or more until fork tender and then serve it with mayonnaise.

Creamy Chicken Soup

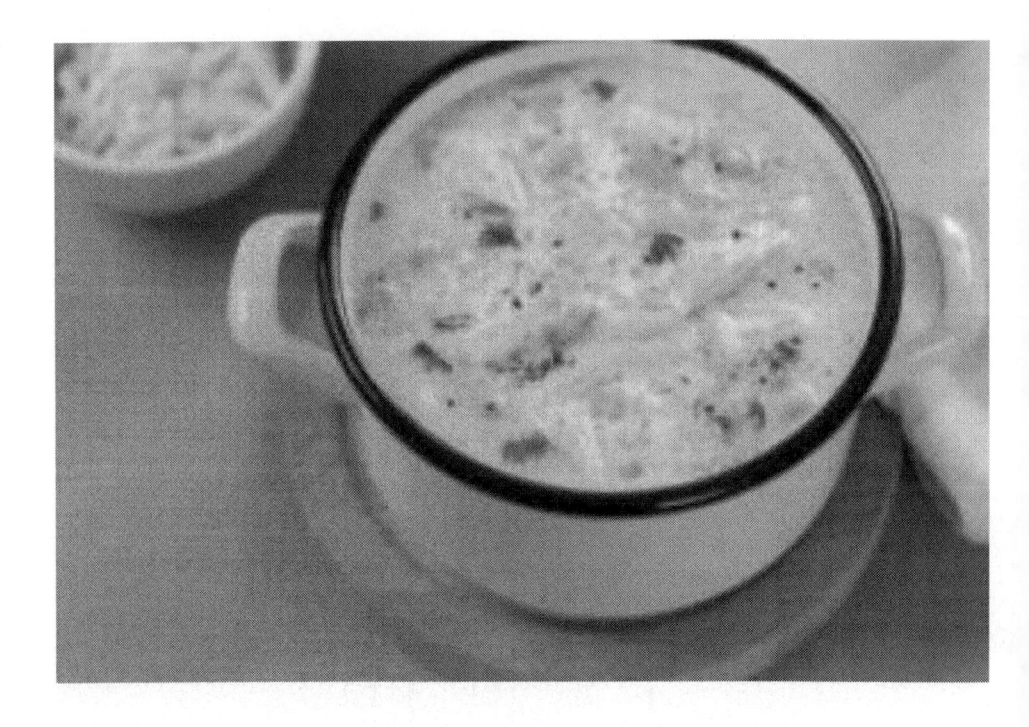

Nutrition Facts Per Serving

Calories	Fats	Proteins	Carbohydrates
647	47.4	50.1	4.9

Ingredients

Serves	1	2	3	4	5	6	7	8
Chicken breast, pasteurized, large	1	2	3	4	5	6	7	8
Cream cheese, softened, cubed, ounces	2	4	6	8	10	12	14	16
Butter, unsalted, tablespoon	1	2	3	4	5	6	7	8
Heavy cream, full-fat, tablespoon	2	4	6	8	10	12	14	16
Chicken broth, pasteurized, ounces	2	4	6	8	10	12	14	16
Italian seasoning, teaspoon	1	2	3	4	5	6	7	8
Salt, by taste								

Instructions

1. Place the chicken in a medium pot, pour in water, place it over medium heat, and cook it for 12 to 15 minutes until tender.
2. Transfer the chicken to a cutting board, shred it, and then reserve the broth.
3. Return the pot over medium heat, add butter, let it melt, add the shredded chicken, and then cook it for 2 minutes until warmed.
4. Add the cheese, salt, and Italian seasoning and then cook for 2 minutes until the cheese melts.
5. Pour in the broth, add the cream, stir until smooth, and then bring the soup to a boil.
6. Then switch heat to medium-low level and simmer the soup for 3 minutes until thickened.
7. Serve straight away.

Cheesy Chicken Stuffed Bell Pepper

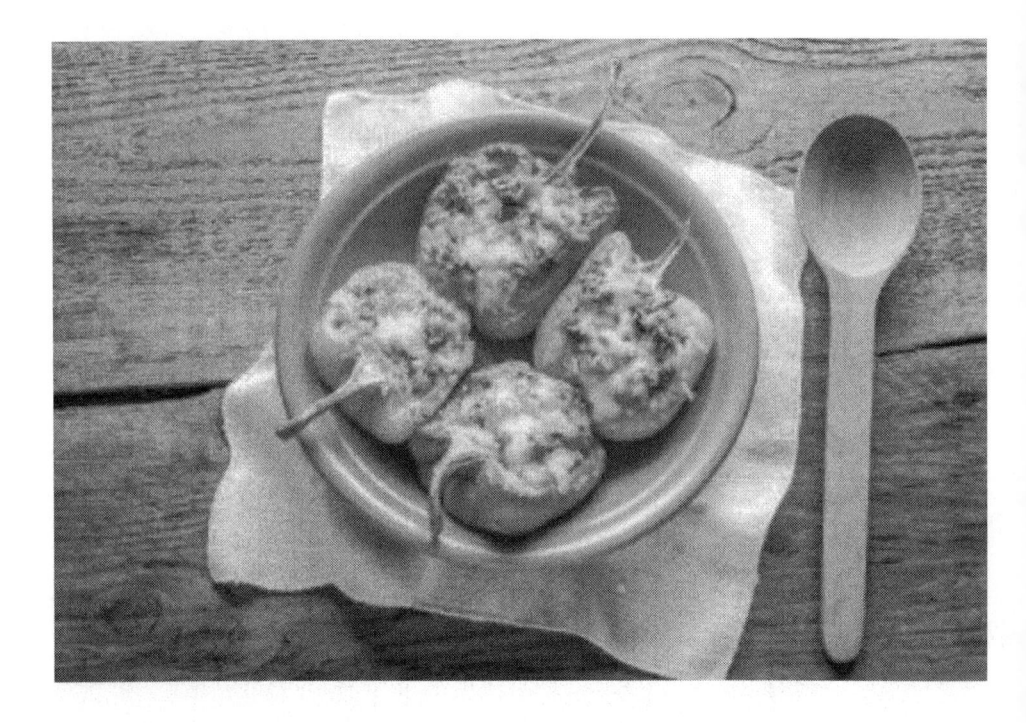

Nutrition Facts Per Serving

Calories	Fats	Proteins	Carbohydrates
341	25	24.7	4.3

Ingredients

Serves	1	2	3	4	5	6	7	8
Ground chicken, pasteurized, ounces	3	6	9	12	15	18	21	24
Bell pepper, medium, cored	1	2	3	4	5	6	7	8
Cream cheese, full-fat, softened, ounces	2	4	6	8	10	12	14	16
Cheddar cheese, grated, full-fat, tablespoon	2	4	6	8	10	12	14	16
Avocado oil, teaspoon	1	2	3	4	5	6	7	8
Paprika, by taste								
Salt, by taste								
Black pepper, by taste								

Instructions

1. Switch on the oven, then set it to 350 degrees F, and let it preheat.
2. In the meantime, place the oil in a medium skillet pan over medium heat and when hot, add the chicken to it.
3. Season with salt, black pepper, and paprika, stir until combined, and then cook it for 8 to 10 minutes until nicely browned and cooked. Next, set aside until required.
4. Remove the top from the bell pepper, remove its core and seeds, and then place it on a parchment-lined baking sheet.
5. Spray the avocado oil over the bell pepper and then bake for 6 minutes.
6. Then spoon the chicken mixture into the bell pepper, and then top with cream cheese. Finally, sprinkle with cheddar cheese.
7. Place the prepared bell pepper under the broiler and then cook for 3 minutes until the cheese melts and becomes golden brown.
8. Serve immediately.

Beef and Spinach Sliders

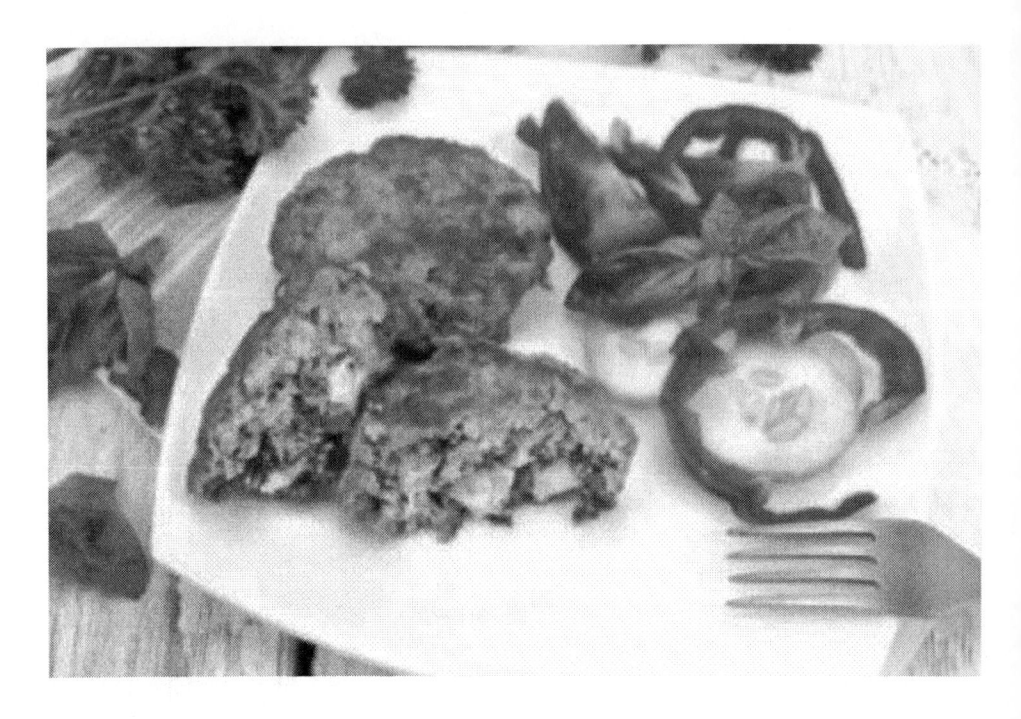

Nutrition Facts Per Serving

Calories	Fats	Proteins	Carbohydrates
414	31.7	31.1	1

Ingredients

Serves	1	2	3	4	5	6	7	8
Chopped spinach, tablespoons	2	4	6	8	10	12	14	16
Ground beef, grass-fed, ounces	4	8	12	16	20	24	28	32
Garlic powder, teaspoon	1	2	3	4	5	6	7	8
Avocado oil, tablespoon	1	2	3	4	5	6	7	8
Lettuce leaf, large	1	2	3	4	5	6	7	8
Salt, by taste								
Black pepper, by taste								

Instructions

1. Place the beef in a medium bowl and then add the spinach, garlic powder, salt, and black pepper.
2. Stir until well combined and then shape the mixture into evenly sized patties.
3. Place the oil in a frying pan, place it over medium heat and when hot, add patties and cook for 5 to 7 minutes per side until golden brown and cooked.
4. When done, place the patties on the lettuce leaf, roll them like a wrap, and then serve.

Basil Stuffed Chicken

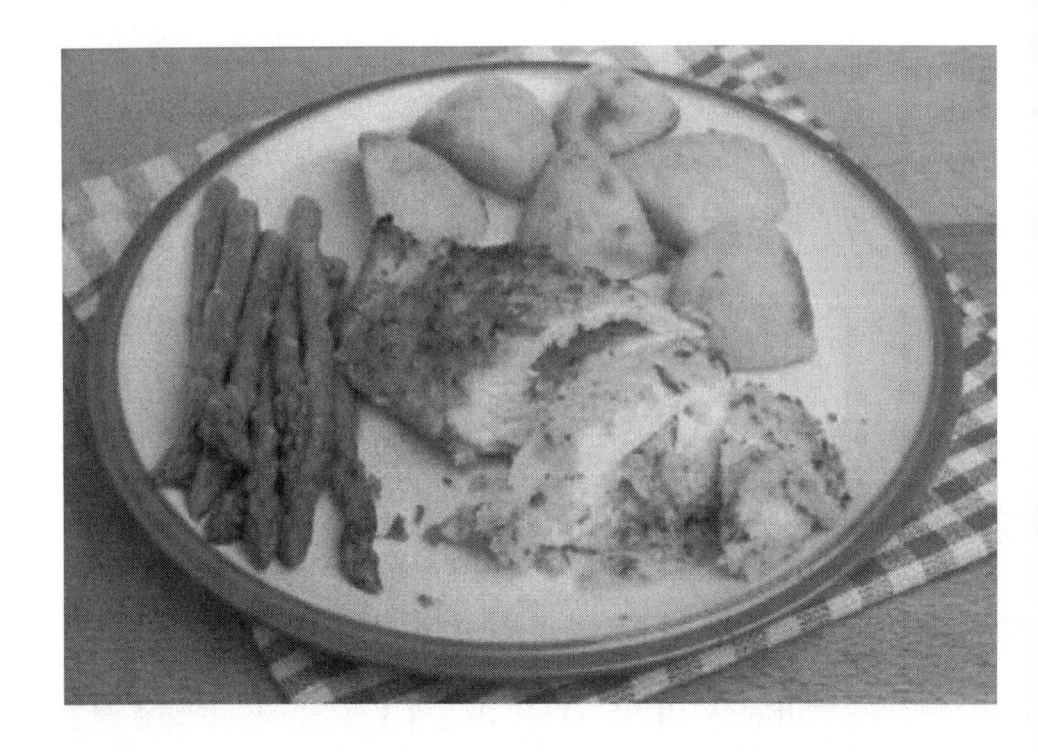

Nutrition Facts Per Serving

Calories	Fats	Proteins	Carbohydrates
413	24.8	46.5	1

Ingredients

Serves	1	2	3	4	5	6	7	8
Chicken breast, large	1	2	3	4	5	6	7	8
Minced garlic, teaspoon	¼	½	¾	1	1¼	1½	1¾	2
Dried basil, teaspoon	1	2	3	4	5	6	7	8
Cream cheese, full-fat, softened, tablespoon	1	2	3	4	5	6	7	8
Mozzarella cheese, full-fat, grated	1	2	3	4	5	6	7	8
Avocado oil, tablespoon	1	2	3	4	5	6	7	8
Salt, by taste								
Black pepper, by taste								

Instructions

1. Switch on the oven, then set it to 375 degrees F, and let it preheat.
2. In the meantime, place garlic in a small bowl, add cream cheese, basil, and mozzarella cheese, and stir until mixed.
3. Make a pocket in the chicken breast, stuff it with the cream cheese mixture, and then secure it with a toothpick.
4. Brush the oil on both sides of chicken, season with salt and black pepper, and then place it on a foil-lined baking sheet.
5. Bake the stuffed chicken for 10 minutes per side until cooked tendered. Finally, serve.

Chicken and Coconut Curry

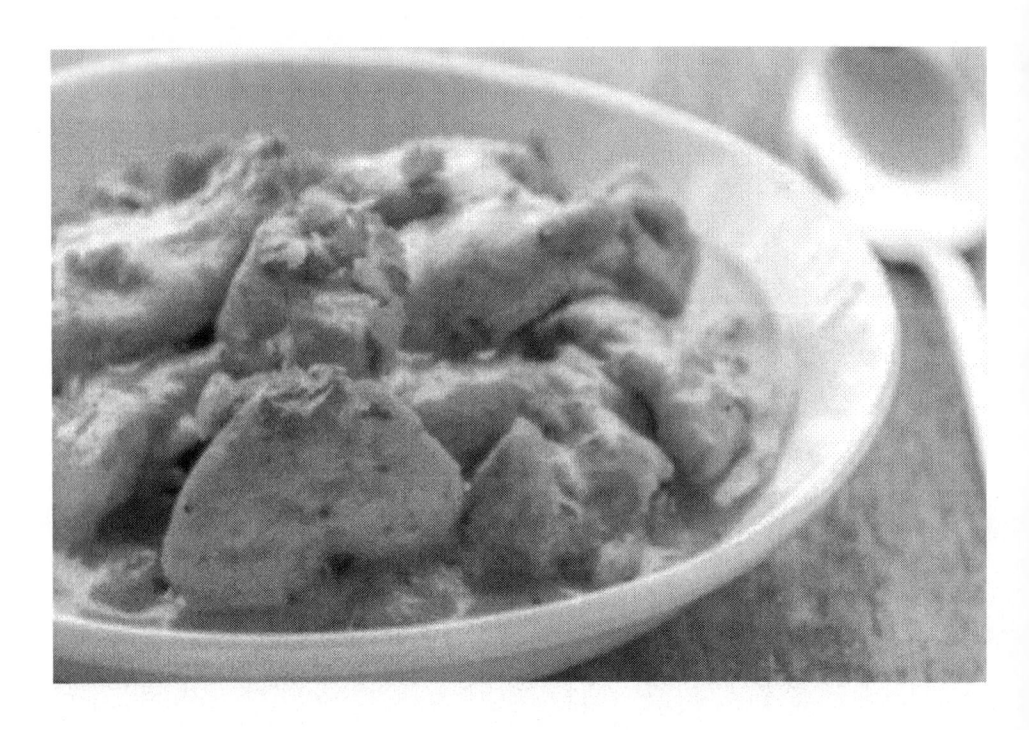

Nutrition Facts Per Serving

Calories	Fats	Proteins	Carbohydrates
375	21.7	44.1	0.9

Ingredients

Serves	1	2	3	4	5	6	7	8
Chicken breast, pasteurized	1	2	3	4	5	6	7	8
Garlic powder, teaspoon	½	1	1½	2	2½	3	3½	4
Curry powder, teaspoon	1	2	3	4	5	6	7	8
Avocado oil, tablespoon	1	2	3	4	5	6	7	8
Coconut milk, full-fat, unsweetened, cup	½	1	1½	2	2½	3	3½	4
Salt, by taste								
Black pepper, by taste								

Instructions

1. Cut the chicken into cubes, place them in a medium bowl, and season with salt and black pepper.
2. Place the oil in a medium saucepan, place it over medium heat and when hot, add the seasoned chicken, and cook for 4 to 5 minutes per side until golden brown.
3. In the meantime, pour the milk in a bowl and then stir in the curry powder.
4. When the chicken has browned, pour the coconut milk mixture into the pan and bring it to a simmer.
5. Then switch the heat to medium-low level and continue simmering for 5 minutes until thoroughly cooked.
6. Serve directly.

Herbed Steaks

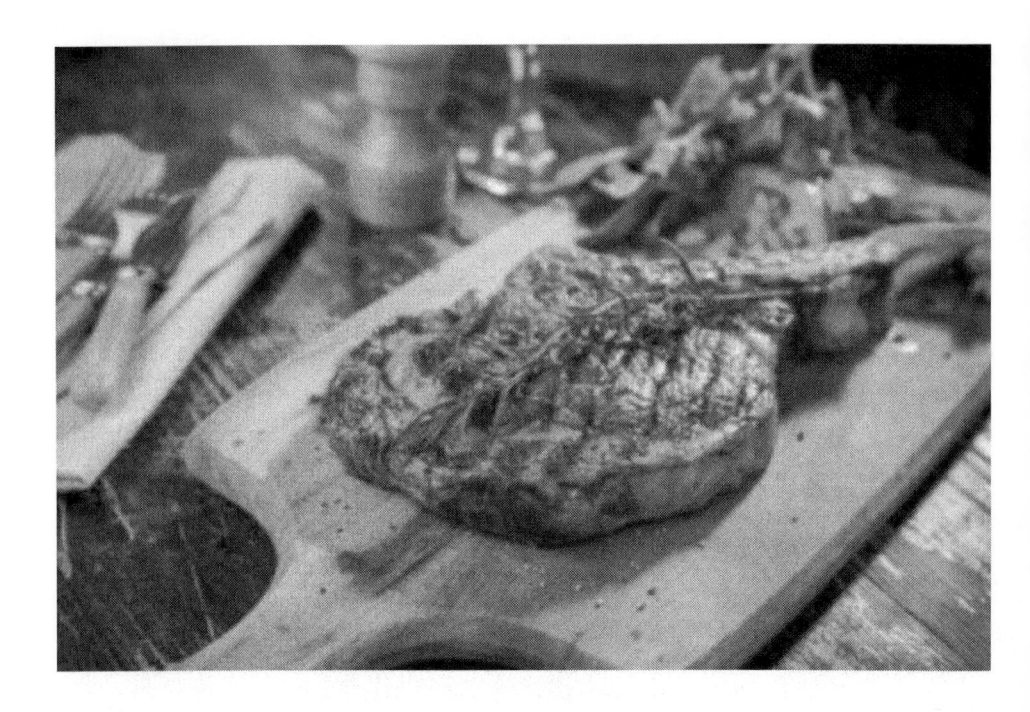

Nutrition Facts Per Serving

Calories	Fats	Proteins	Carbohydrates
426	31.7	34.1	1.1

Ingredients

Serves	1	2	3	4	5	6	7	8
Beef sirloin steak, grass-fed	1	2	3	4	5	6	7	8
Lime juice, tablespoon	1	2	3	4	5	6	7	8
Dried rosemary, teaspoon	1	2	3	4	5	6	7	8
Dried basil, teaspoon	1	2	3	4	5	6	7	8
Avocado oil, tablespoon	3	6	9	12	15	18	21	24
Salt, by taste								
Black pepper, by taste								

Instructions

1. Place 2 tablespoons oil in a shallow dish, add lime juice, and then stir until combined.
2. Season the steak with garlic powder, add to the lime juice mixture, toss until coated, and then let it marinate for 20 minutes.
3. Then add the remaining oil on a griddle pan, place it over medium-high heat and when hot, place steak in it.
4. Cook the steak for 4 to 8 minutes per side until cooked to desired doneness and then let it rest for 5 minutes.
5. Cut the steak into slices and then serve.

Pork Cutlets

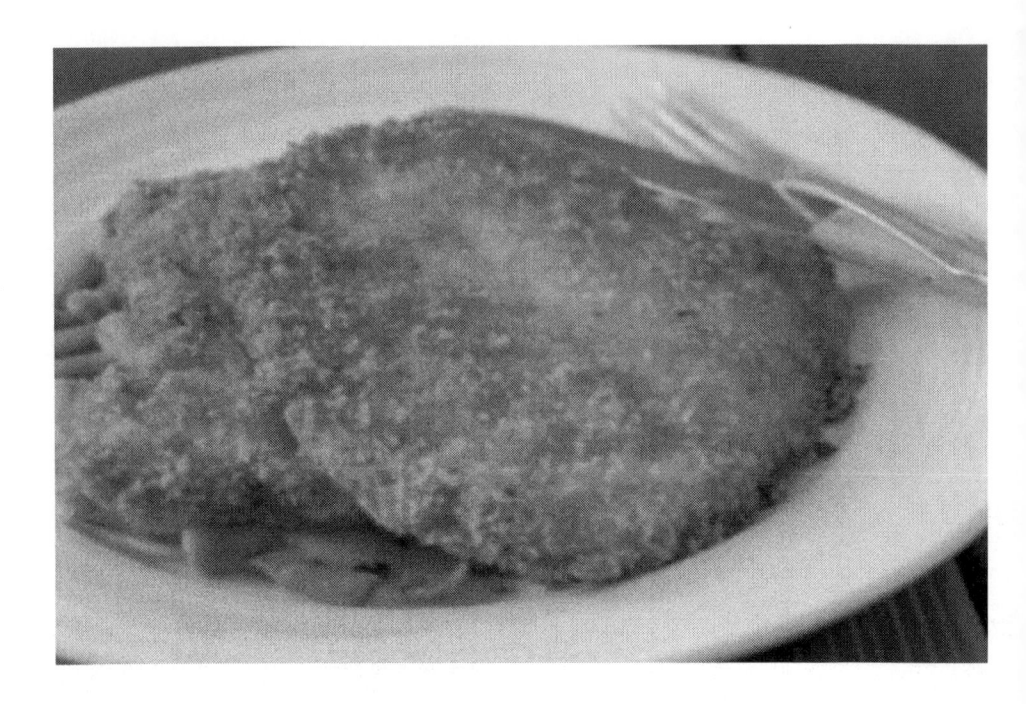

Nutrition Facts Per Serving

Calories	Fats	Proteins	Carbohydrates
678	50.5	49.2	6.8

Ingredients

Serves	1	2	3	4	5	6	7	8
Ground pork, pasteurized, ounces	4	8	12	16	20	24	28	32
Egg, pasteurized	1	2	3	4	5	6	7	8
Coconut flour, tablespoon	2	4	6	8	10	12	14	16
Parmesan cheese, grated, full-fat, tablespoon	4	8	12	16	20	24	28	32
Avocado oil, tablespoon	1	2	3	4	5	6	7	8
Salt, by taste								
Black pepper, by taste								

Instructions

1. Place the ground pork in a medium bowl, add cheese, salt, black pepper, and egg, and then stir until combined.
2. Shape the pork mixture into two evenly size patties and then refrigerate them for 30 minutes.
3. Then place the oil in a skillet pan, place it over medium heat and let it heat until hot.
4. Dredge the patties in coconut flour until coated, add them to the pan and then cook for 5 to 8 minutes per side until cooked and nicely browned.
5. Serve immediately.

Pork Chops with Mushrooms

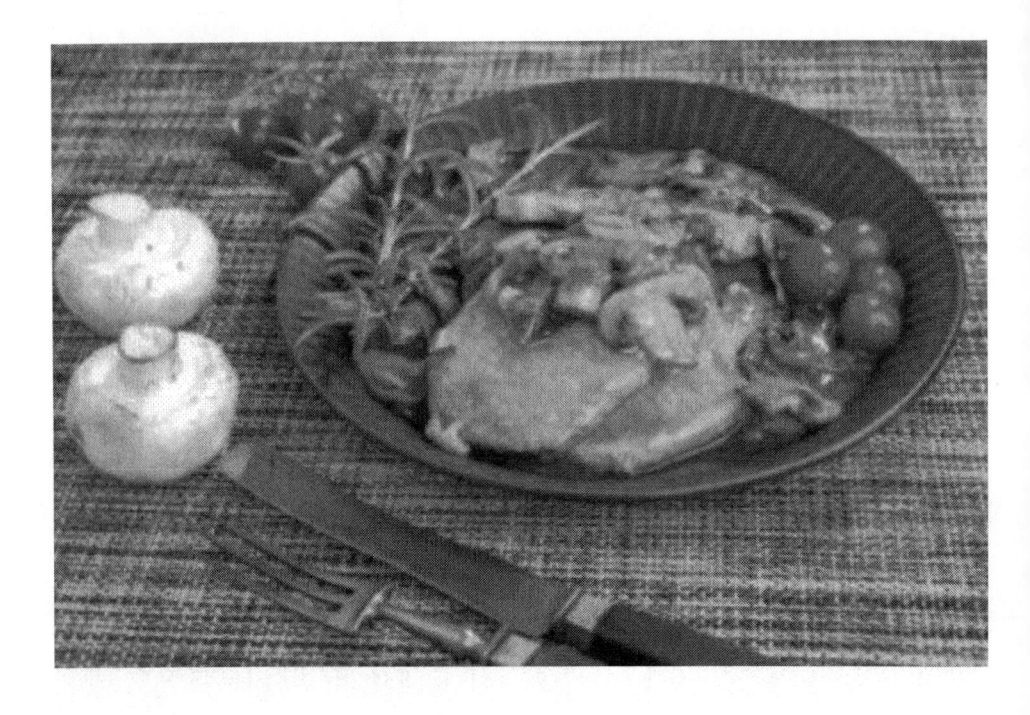

Nutrition Facts Per Serving

Calories	Fats	Proteins	Carbohydrates
628	53	36.1	1.6

Ingredients

Serves	1	2	3	4	5	6	7	8
Pork chop, pasteurized, about 4 ounces	1	2	3	4	5	6	7	8
Sliced mushrooms, ounces	2	4	6	8	10	12	14	16
Avocado oil, tablespoon	1	2	3	4	5	6	7	8
Butter, unsalted, tablespoon	2	4	6	8	10	12	14	16
Water, tablespoon	2	4	6	8	10	12	14	16
Salt, by taste								
Paprika, by taste								

Instructions

1. Place the pork chop in a shallow dish and then season it with salt and black pepper.
2. Place the oil in a skillet pan, place it over medium heat and when hot, add pork chop and then cook it for 4 minutes per side until nicely browned.
3. When done, transfer the chop to a plate, add butter into the pan and let it melt.
4. Add the mushrooms, season with salt and paprika, and then cook for 3 to 4 minutes until tender.
5. Add water, stir until mixed, bring it to simmer, then add the pork chop and continue cooking for 3 minutes until done.
6. Serve immediately.

Cocoa Rubbed Pork

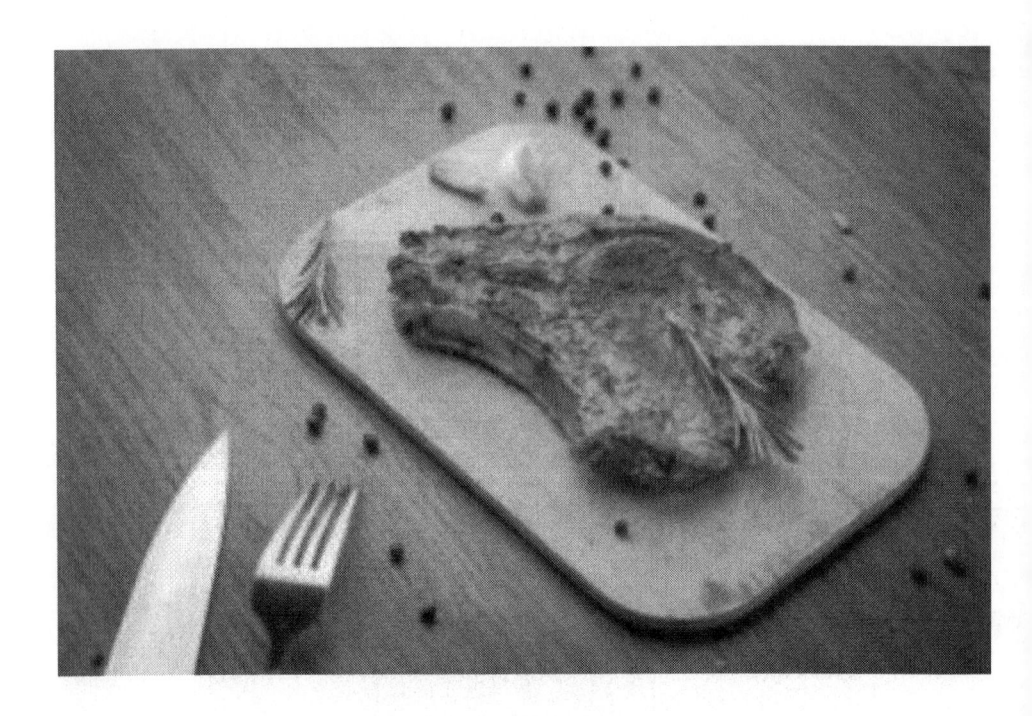

Nutrition Facts Per Serving

Calories	Fats	Proteins	Carbohydrates
375	25.4	35.6	0.9

Ingredients

Serves	1	2	3	4	5	6	7	8
Pork chop, pasteurized, about 4 ounces	1	2	3	4	5	6	7	8
Ground coriander, teaspoon	½	1	1½	2	2½	3	3½	4
Ground nutmeg, teaspoon	½	1	1½	2	2½	3	3½	4
Cocoa powder, unsweetened, tablespoon	1	2	3	4	5	6	7	8
Avocado oil, tablespoon	1	2	3	4	5	6	7	8
Salt, by taste								
Black pepper, by taste								

Instructions

1. Switch on the oven, then set it to 400 degrees F and let it preheat.
2. Place the coriander in a small bowl, add salt, black pepper, nutmeg, and cocoa powder and then stir until mixed.
3. Rub this spice mixture on both sides of the pork chop until coated.
4. Place oil in a skillet pan and when hot, add the pork chops and then cook for 2 minutes per side until beginning to brown.
5. Bake the pork chop in the pan for 5 minutes per side until tender and cooked and then serve.

Conclusion

Congratulations on deciding that you deserve better. Everyone deserves to feel healthy and happy. Everyone deserves to have a body that they are comfortable with. With keto, you've taken your first step through the door towards bettering yourself and your life. This journey won't always be smooth, since you may stumble at times, but as long as you persevere and keep trying your hardest, you'll always come out on top.

All in all, follow your plan step-by-step, keep your goals in mind, and whenever you need some guidance, feel free to return to this book. You have every tool you need to change your life for the better. Your motivation and drive that has taken you to the end of this book will fulfill whatever goals you have. Take the recipes, advice, knowledge, and inevitable results from this book into the world with you and flaunt them for all to see. You've earned it for the bravery in deciding to make a positive change!

References

Brehm, B. J., Seeley, R. J., Daniels, S. R., & D'Alessio, D. A. (2003). A Randomized Trial Comparing a Very Low Carbohydrate Diet and a Calorie-Restricted Low Fat Diet on Body Weight and Cardiovascular Risk Factors in Healthy Women. *The Journal of Clinical Endocrinology & Metabolism, 88*(4), 1617–1623. https://doi.org/10.1210/jc.2002-021480

Clarke, C. (2013a, October 20). *How To Transition To The Keto Diet [5 Critical Steps]*. Ruled Me. https://www.ruled.me/transition-to-keto-diet/

Clarke, C. (2013b, October 27). *Keto Sweetener Guide: Best & Worst [Sucrolose, Stevia, Erythritol]*. Ruled Me. https://www.ruled.me/keto-diet-plan-best-and-worst-sweeteners/

Eenfeldt, A. (2019, March 19). *Ketogenic diet foods – what to eat*. Diet Doctor. https://www.dietdoctor.com/low-carb/keto/foods

Emory University Health Sciences Center. (2005, October 15). *Ketogenic Diet Prevents Seizures By Enhancing Brain Energy Production, Increasing Neuron Stability*. ScienceDaily. https://www.sciencedaily.com/releases/2005/11/051114220938.htm#:~:text=New%20studies%20show%20that%20the

Fine, E. J., Segal-Isaacson, C. J., Feinman, R. D., Herszkopf, S., Romano, M. C., Tomuta, N., Bontempo, A. F., Negassa, A., & Sparano, J. A. (2012). Targeting insulin inhibition as a metabolic therapy in advanced cancer: a pilot safety and feasibility dietary trial in 10 patients. *Nutrition (Burbank, Los Angeles County, Calif.), 28*(10), 1028–1035. https://doi.org/10.1016/j.nut.2012.05.001

Frey, M. (2020, May 16). *How the Ketogenic Diet Compares to Others.* Verywell Fit. https://www.verywellfit.com/how-does-the-ketogenic-diet-compare-to-other-diets-4687538

Harvard T.H. Chan. (2018, May 7). *Diet Review: Ketogenic Diet for Weight Loss.* The Nutrition Source. https://www.hsph.harvard.edu/nutritionsource/healthy-weight/diet-reviews/ketogenic-diet/

Health.gov. (n.d.). *Appendix 2. Estimated Calorie Needs per Day, by Age, Sex, and Physical Activity Level - 2015-2020 Dietary Guidelines | health.gov.* Health.Gov. Retrieved July 28, 2020, from https://health.gov/our-work/food-nutrition/2015-2020-dietary-guidelines/guidelines/appendix-2/

Kubala, J. (2018, August 21). *A Keto Diet Meal Plan and Menu That Can Transform Your Body.* Healthline. https://www.healthline.com/nutrition/keto-diet-meal-plan-and-menu#the-basics

Link, R. (2020, March 17). *Working Out on Keto: All You Need to Know.* Healthline. https://www.healthline.com/nutrition/working-out-on-keto#best-exercises-for-keto

Westman, E. C., Yancy, W. S., Mavropoulos, J. C., Marquart, M., & McDuffie, J. R. (2008). The effect of a low-carbohydrate, ketogenic diet versus a low-glycemic index diet on glycemic control in type 2 diabetes mellitus. *Nutrition & Metabolism, 5*(1). https://doi.org/10.1186/1743-7075-5-36

Printed in Great Britain
by Amazon